Diabetic Foot Care

Diabetic Foot Care

Case Studies in Clinical Management

Alethea Foster and Michael Edmonds
The Diabetic Foot Clinic, King's College Hospital, London, UK

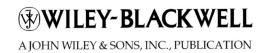

A JOHN WILEY & SONS, INC., PUBLICATION

Library of Congress Cataloguing-in-Publication Data

Foster, Alethea V. M.
    Diabetic foot care : case studies in clinical management / Alethea Foster and Michael Edmonds.
        p. ; cm.
    Includes index.
    ISBN 978-0-470-99823-6 (cloth)
    1. Foot–Diseases–Treatment–Case studies.   2. Diabetes–Complications–Treatment–Case studies.
3. Foot manifestations of general diseases–Case studies.
I. Edmonds, M. E.   II. Title.
    [DNLM: 1. Diabetic Foot–therapy–Case Reports. 2. Diabetic Foot–diagnosis–Case Reports.
WK 835 F754d 2010]
    RC951.F674 2010
    616.6′1–dc22
                                                                2010025371

A catalogue record for this book is available from the British Library.

This book is published in the following electronic formats: ePDF 9780470682937; Wiley Online Library 9780470682944

Set in 10.5/12.5pt, Minion by Thomson Digital, Noida, India.
Printed and bound in Singapore by Markono Print Media Pte Ltd.

First impression   2011

*This book is dedicated to all our living patients,
as a tribute to men and women of remarkable
fortitude and courage,*

*and is also dedicated to the memory of our patients
who have died valiantly fighting diabetes and who have
shown us how diabetes can be a killer*

Contents

Acknowledgements

We are grateful to colleagues past and present, who include: Simon Fraser, Huw Walters, Mary Blundell, Cathy Eaton, Mark Greenhill, Susie Spencer, Maureen McColgan-Bates, Mel Doxford, Sally Wilson, Adora Hatrapal, E Maelor Thomas, Mick Morris, Joh Philpott-Howard, Jim Wade, Andrew Hay, Robert Lewis, Anne- Marie Ryan, Irina Mantey, Robert Hills, Rachel Ben-Salem, Muriel Buxton-Thomas, Mazin Al-Janabi, Dawn Hurley, Stephanie Amiel, Stephen Thomas, Daniela Pitei, Paul Baskerville, Anthony Giddings, Irving Benjamin, Mark Myerson, Paul Sidhu, Joydeep Sinha, Patricia Wallace, Gillian Cavell, Lesley Boys, Magdi Hanna, Sue Peat, Colin Roberts, David Goss, Colin Deane, Sue Snowdon, Ana Grenfell, TimCundy, Pat Ascott, Lindis Richards, Kate Spicer, Debbie Broome, Liz Hampton, Timothy Jemmott, Michelle Buckley, Rosalind Phelan, Maggie Boase, Maria Back, Julie Lambert, Avril Witherington, Daniel Rajan, Hisham Rashid, Ghulam Mufti, Karen Fairbairn, Ian Eltringham, Nina Petrova, Lindy Begg, Barbara Wall, Mark O'Brien, Sacha Andrews, Barry Pike, Jane Preece, Briony Sloper, Christian Pankhurst, Jim Beaumont, Matthew McShane, Tim Cooney, Lin Pan , Cheryl Clark, Marcello Perez, Nicholas Cooley, Paul Bains, Patricia Yerbury, Charlotte Biggs, Anna Korzon Burakowska, David Ross, Jason Wilkins, David Evans, Dean Huang, Carol Gayle, David Hopkins, Rif Malik, Keith Jones, Bob Edmondson, Enid Joseph, Karen Reid, David Williams , Doris Agyemang-Duah, Jennifer Tremlett, Venu Kavarthapu, Om Lahoti and Mark Phillips, Paula Gardiner, Ian Alejandro, Barbara Chirara, Victoria Morris, Hany Zayed, Paul Donohoe and Sui PhinKon and two great stalwarts of the Foot Clinic, Peter Watkins and the late David Pyke.

The Podiatry Managers and Community Podiatrists from Lambeth, Southwark and Lewisham have also contributed greatly to the work of the Foot Clinic at King's over many years.

We are particularly grateful for the advice of the members of the Dermatology Department, Anthony du Vivier, Daniel Creamer, Claire Fuller, Elisabeth Higgins, Sarah MacFarlane, Rachel Morris-Jones and Saqib Bashir.

We also are also thankful to Stephen and Audrey Edmonds and to Nina Petrova for technical help with the production of the manuscript.

We give special thanks to Yvonne Bartlett, Alex Dionysiou, David Langdon, Lucy Wallace, Margaret Delaney and Moira Lovell from the Department of Medical Photography at King's.

We are particularly grateful to Fiona Woods Project editor, STM books, Wiley-Blackwell and Sarah Abdul Karim, Production Editor, Content Management, Wiley-Blackwell and Aparajita Srivastava, Senior Project Manager, Thomson Digital for their patience and help.

Introduction

In this book, we describe cases from the King's Diabetic Foot Clinic archive, most of which have not previously been described in any of our books. We have always believed that there are lessons to be learned from every single patient, and if those lessons can be passed on to other health care professionals through this book then the patients described will not have suffered or died in vain. Each patient is unique and complex and a wonderful learning resource.

The book is aimed at all health care professionals who care for or come into contact with diabetic patients. By reading these case reports we hope that all these professionals should come to understand the subtleties and complexities of diabetic foot presentations, and in particular the general points about diabetic foot patients, namely, that patients with diabetic foot problems quickly reach the point of no return and often have multiple co-morbidities which affect the progress of their foot condition. Indeed, the exacerbation of their foot problem often aggravates their co-morbidities. However, close medical attention to their co-morbidities both in the Diabetic Foot Clinic and on the Hospital wards can lead to a positive outcome and an improvement in their foot condition. The underlying principles of diabetic foot care are early diagnosis and intervention and meticulous follow-up. All health care professionals should be aware of this.

Patients often have other co-morbidities that contribute to their pathogenesis of the diabetic foot, for example, renal failure. This can then be affected by the diabetic foot lesion with worsening renal failure especially in the presence of infection, and the renal status will also impact on their overall progress.

Within these case studies we have tried to get across the feeling of how it is in the real world, trying to manage diabetic foot patients with long-term, end-stage diabetes, within the Diabetic Foot Clinic and on the Hospital wards. We describe the failures as well as the successes, the frustrations as well as the achievements and the camaraderie of working within a multidisciplinary team of like-minded and dedicated practitioners

The patients described are difficult patients and vulnerable patients and managing them well is hard work. Complex medical and psychosocial factors lead to difficulties and barriers. By describing our clinical experiences, the problems we and our patients have faced, and the lessons we have learned over the years in managing these unpredictable patients with multiple co-morbidities, we hope it will become clear that these patients need to be managed within an expert environment. Sometimes the only way to achieve healing is with advanced techniques. The support of a multidisciplinary team is essential: the combined skills of vascular surgeon and interventional radiologist, orthopaedic surgeon microbiologist, dermatologist, psychologist, physician, podiatrist, nurse and orthotist are often needed. Although we have always promoted the importance of basic foot care and preventive education, there is sometimes also a need for access to advanced techniques to achieve healing.

We describe the multidisciplinary and supportive approach to patients that we use at King's to try to keep patients out of trouble. All diabetic foot patients with severe problems that we have seen at King's had one or more of the following four problems:

Neuropathy,

Ischaemia,

Charcot's osteoarthropathy

Renal impairment,

and this book is broken into four main sections devoted to those four categories of patient. There are some areas of overlap in the case histories: some patients have spent periods of their diabetic lives in all of the sections, progressing from neuropathy to the development of Charcot's osteoarthropathy and on to neuroischaemia and eventual renal failure.

The same principles of care recur time and time again. First and foremost is the need to classify and stage the foot, and we use our King's Simple Staging System, which follows the diabetic foot along the road to amputation, and can be used as a framework for organising care. It goes as follows:

First we classify the foot as neuropathic or neuroischaemic. We then stage the foot.

- Stage 1   The normal foot
- Stage 2   The high risk foot (with one or more of the following: neuropathy, ischaemia, deformity, swelling, callus)
- Stage 3   The ulcerated foot
- Stage 4   The infected foot
- Stage 5   The necrotic foot
- Stage 6   The unsalvageable foot

We have described this Simple Staging System to manage patients in our previous diabetic foot books. The principles of management according to the Simple Staging System have been applied to every patient in the book – it has become second nature to us to use this tool - but we have not elaborated on this in detail with every patient case as doing that would become repetitious and tedious. We have tried to stress the most relevant and interesting points in each case without labouring the points that have already been covered in other case histories.

In our selection of case histories we have tried to illustrate new developments in each area, over the 29 years that the King's Diabetic Foot Clinic has existed, and also the problems that can arise when new techniques are applied to diabetic patients. The cases in this book illustrate the 'King's Approach', and the same principles of care recur time and time again: the importance of catching problems early, the aggressive management of infection, never underestimating apparently small problems, especially when they occur in a foot with ischaemia or a patient with renal impairment, the gradual building up of a relationship of trust over many years, and the constant search for potential problems which can be prevented, delayed or de-toothed with education or a change in the management or just a little compromise on either side. Lastly, the involvement of patients and their families in the clinical decisions made is, we believe, essential to successful management of the high-risk diabetic foot: the patients with supportive, caring, observant families do best.

Although the foot problems are serious, with greater overall mortality than cancer of the colon, and at least fifty percent of the patients described are in the last few months or years of their lives, nonetheless, the life of the diabetic foot patient can be extended and their happiness and mobility optimised by good foot care.

Alethea Foster
London, 2010   **Michael Edmonds**

Glossary of terms

Throughout this book we refer to:

ABPI	Ankle brachial pressure index
bd	twice daily
BMD	Bone mineral density
CAPD	Continuous ambulatory peritoneal dialysis
CROW	Charcot restraint orthotic walker
CRP	C-reactive protein
CVA	Cerebrovascular accident
EMG	Electromyography
ESBL	*Extended sensitivity beta lactamase*
IM	Intramuscular
INR	International Normalised Ratio
IV	Intravenous
MRA	Magnetic Resonance Angiography
MRI	Magnetic Resonance Imaging
MRSA	Methicillin resistant staphylococcus aureus
MSU	Mid stream specimen of urine
PICC	Peripherally inserted central catheter
PTBWRO	Patellar-tendon-bearing weight-relieving orthosis
qds	four times daily
tds	three times daily
VAC	Vacuum assisted closure
VPT	Vibration perception threshold measured at the apex of the big toe
WBC	White blood count

1
Neuropathic Case Studies

1.1 Introduction

In the past we have often described the neuropathic foot as a 'forgiving' foot, and there is little doubt that of the four main categories of patients – neuropaths, neuroischaemics, renals and Charcots – described in this book it is the neuropathic patients who do the best. It is, however, important never to underestimate the problems of the diabetic patient with neuropathy, which is a devastating deficit. In many of these patients, neuropathy affects other anatomical systems such as the cardiovascular, gastrointestinal and urogenital systems, and not just their feet and legs, and as a result they are incredibly frail and vulnerable, with greatly increased susceptibility to infections and other insults. When managing the neuropathic patient with foot problems, particular regard must be paid to all these susceptibilities and vulnerabilities. It is often said of these patients with neuropathic feet "Good pulses, not ischaemic, not in trouble" – but the neuropathic patient is actually very fragile and may rapidly develop severe problems and therefore can get into trouble very quickly.

In choosing sections for this chapter, we have included those that substantially affect the patient with diabetic neuropathic feet: highlighting first the role of infection, the "great destroyer", which is a real mask of Janus, putting on so many different and deceptive faces in the diabetic patient (a theme that is repeated in every chapter). Second comes the effect of neuropathy in conjunction with other co-morbidities that are present in the neuropathic patient. Third, we look at the effect of reconstruction of the deformed or unstable neuropathic foot. Fourth, we consider the significance of psychological factors, and finally, the importance of long term care.

The diabetic foot with neuropathy is very susceptible to traumatic damage, leading to a break in the skin, which then acts as a portal of entry of infection. Colleagues from Africa and India have frequently described devastating infections that rapidly destroy the neuropathic foot. Now that London is an international city we too now see patients with horrendous infections, including those who have travelled from Africa and India, and this type of rapidly destructive infection is described in this section. In temperate climes as well as tropical ones, there is increased susceptibility of the diabetic neuropathic foot to

Diabetic Foot Care: Case Studies in Clinical Management   Alethea Foster and Michael Edmonds
© 2011 John Wiley & Sons, Ltd.

infection, and we see very severe infections where the serum C-reactive protein (CRP) can be above 400 mg/l. Furthermore, when a neuropathic patient becomes systemically unwell then almost certainly the infection is very severe. We have also learnt that diabetic neuropathic patients are prone not only to foot infections but also to devastating infections elsewhere in the body.

Aggressive treatment of infection is important, starting with wide spectrum antibiotic therapy and then targeting therapy according to bacteria isolated. It is important to have a working knowledge of the principal bacteria and their local antibiotic sensitivities, including awareness of the prevalence of resistant organisms. However, in every patient, individual sensitivities of each organism isolated on culture should be sought to guide rational antibiotic therapy. There should be close co-operation between the microbiology laboratory and the diabetic foot service. Furthermore, antibiotic therapy should be accompanied by debridement of infective and necrotic tissue. When patients present with severe infection they need expert medical treatment including careful fluid replacement. Perioperative problems are common: in the early days of the Diabetic Foot Clinic we saw a patient who suffered respiratory arrest on codeine tablets and had to be temporarily ventilated.

We have also come to learn that diabetic neuropathic patients are frail vulnerable patients and we have also considered the impact that neuropathy and also co-morbidities can have on the diabetic patient. Peripheral neuropathy itself produces a major deficit of sensation in the lower limbs. It impairs proprioception and patients with neuropathy become very unsteady, and falls and associated traumatic lesions are common. Other complications, including postural hypotension and hypoglycaemic episodes without any warnings, make accidents even more likely. Neuropathy is a devastating deficit, and it is not just the feet and legs that are affected. The diabetic patient with a neuropathic ulcer will usually have evidence of nerve damage elsewhere. Autonomic neuropathy may affect the heart, gastrointestinal system and bladder. Damage to the nerve supply of the heart can lead to silent ischaemia and silent myocardial infarction. We have seen cases of sudden death in young, apparently robust neuropathic patients who had no peripheral vascular disease. There may be poor neurological control of ventilation leading to sleep apnoea and also susceptibility to pulmonary infections. In addition to neuropathy, co-morbidities may include poor vision through diabetic retinopathy and cataract.

Key principles to remember are that neuropathic patients may become destabilised by ulceration and sepsis and that neuropathic ulcers may present in various ways, often as medical emergencies with not only severe, rapidly progressing infections but also considerable metabolic upset.

Diabetic neuropathic patients who present with ulceration and infection often have deformity of the foot that has precipitated the initial ulceration. Such patients often need surgical debridement and in addition can benefit at the same time from surgical correction. If our early neuropathic patients seen in the 1980s and 90s developed severe deformity of the feet, the standard approach was to accommodate such deformity with appropriate footwear, but it is now possible to correct the deformity surgically as well as heal the ulcers.

In addition to the impact of other co-morbidities, psychological problems are also very important. Many diabetic foot patients, when they are first referred to us, are deeply fearful, believing that they face inevitable amputation. The majority of patients rapidly gain confidence once they feel that they have found a safe haven where rapid and appropriate treatment will always be available. Patients build up relationships with the staff of the Diabetic Foot Clinic over many years, and even patients who do not always follow advice or do not always accept treatment are still cared for. However, some patients have concurrent psychological problems and remain deeply suspicious and often unwilling to accept care. Furthermore, there may be problems of self-delusion, when patients convince themselves that devastating foot infections are trivial.

We emphasize the need for long term management in a specialist Diabetic Foot Clinic for these patients.

Each diabetic neuropathic patient is unique, always beginning with the assumption that any person with diabetic neuropathy is a very vulnerable patient. It is important to have a thorough long term knowledge and understanding of the patient in order to apply effectively modern techniques for optimal diagnosis and treatment. Although we have always emphasized the need to make a clear distinction between the well perfused neuropathic foot and the neuroischaemic foot, it should never be forgotten that if a classical neuropathic patient lives long enough he is likely eventually to develop ischaemia. All the patients described in the neuroischaemic chapter will have started their diabetic foot lives as neuropathic patients. The diabetic foot is a moving target!

In this chapter we describe 36 cases of neuropathic foot disease. They fall into five main groups.

- Patients with differing presentations of infection and complications of infection.

- Patients with co-morbidities in addition to diabetes and neuropathy impacting on neuropathic foot presentations.

- Patients presenting with neuropathic foot deformity, ulceration and infection, when reconstruction to correct the deformity is carried out as well as surgical debridement for the infection.

- Patients with neuropathic feet in whom psychological factors have impacted on their management.

- Long term patients followed in the Diabetic Foot Clinic with neuropathic foot problems.

1.2 Differing presentations of infection and complications of infection

The first series of cases in this chapter are different presentations of infection because these are the most serious and dramatic problems in the diabetic neuropathic foot. Even a slightly raised body temperature can mark a severe infection with the capacity to deteriorate with alarming rapidity.

Case 1.1   A slightly raised body temperature can be a marker of severe infection, which can lead to collapse within hours

A 40 year old man with Type 2 diabetes for 6 years had proliferative retinopathy and peripheral and autonomic neuropathy. Vibration sensation was absent at both great toes. He sustained plantar blisters on both his feet after walking around the house barefooted on a nylon carpet after soaking in a long hot bath (Figure 1.1a). On the first occasion he was encouraged to rest and take time off work so that the blisters would heal quickly. He did not follow this advice and developed a large neuropathic ulcer on the left forefoot (Stage 3 foot), after which he agreed to rest as much as possible and the ulcer quickly began to heal (Figure 1.1b) and was completely healed in two months. He was reluctant to wear bespoke shoes but agreed to wear trainers. Two further episodes of blistering healed quickly.

However, five years later he developed another large blister on the right foot and attended the Foot Clinic. There was no obvious spreading infection but he had local cellulitis and a body temperature of 37.7 °C and it was decided to admit him (Stage 4 foot).

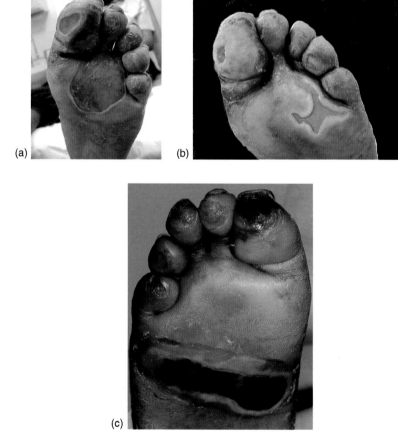

(a)   (b)

(c)

Figure 1.1   (a) Plantar blisters. (b) Healing foot. (c) The foot with necrosis.

He insisted on going home first because he wished to take his car home as it was parked in a hospital car park. He said that he would leave his car at home and ask his brother to bring him to the hospital. He was brought back by his brother later that afternoon. In two hours he had become extremely ill, with a body temperature of 40.2 °C. He was very drowsy and shivering and had a spreading cellulitis. Blood pressure was 90/60 mm Hg. He was admitted at once. He was immediately given quadruple IV antibiotics according to our usual regime of amoxicillin 500 mg tds, flucloxacillin 500 mg qds, metronidazole 500 mg tds and ceftazidime 1 g tds. He was started on IV insulin sliding scale. Blood cultures grew *Staphylococcus aureus* and Group G *Streptococcus* and his IV antibiotics were then rationalised to amoxicillin and flucloxacillin. He was also treated with clindamycin 450 mg qds IV. The CRP on admission was 166.5 mg/l, falling to 104.2 mg/l the next day, 41.8 mg/l after two days and 19.1 mg/l after four days. On admission the white blood count (WBC) was 12.77×10^9/l, with a neutrophilia of 10.66×10^9/l, falling after four days to a WBC of 4.64×10^9/l and neutrophils normal at 2.79×10^9/l. Glycated haemoglobin was 11.7%. The blister developed into an area of necrosis (Figure 1.1c) but this gradually improved. He was discharged after 10 days. After this episode he agreed to check his feet every day and come to the Diabetic Foot Clinic regularly and he has not relapsed.

Learning points

- Systemic symptoms and bacteraemia can develop rapidly from diabetic foot infections. It is very risky to allow any delays in admission, for example when patients wish to go home to collect possessions.

- A high fever, as in this case, is usually indicative of a very severe infection and is associated with a bacteraemia. Blood cultures should be carried out on all diabetic patients with foot infections and a fever, however mild this fever is.

- The clinician should beware of even mild fever as any fever is a sign of a serious infection. However, many diabetic patients do not develop fever even when they have a foot infection.

- Clindamycin was used because the patient had signs of toxicity with high fever and clindamycin is a powerful inhibitor of streptococcal toxin synthesis.

- When using clindamycin it is necessary to be aware of antibiotic-induced colitis, especially in elderly and postoperative patients.

- Serial measurements of falling serum CRP levels can confirm progress in resolving infection.

- *Staphylococcus aureus* is the commonest cause of infection in the diabetic foot and is often accompanied by a streptococcal infection of either Group B or Group G and rarely Group A. These organisms act in synergy and can lead to considerable tissue necrosis because hyaluronidase, produced by the *Streptococcus*, facilitates the spread of toxins produced by the *Staphylococcus*.

Case 1.2   Even if the pedal pulses are strong, necrosis develops when infection is severe

Another common presentation of infection in the neuropathic foot is of gangrene: the diabetic black toe. Previously, necrosis in a diabetic foot with palpable pedal pulses was deemed to be due to "small vessel disease", and the unfortunate patient often found himself on the receiving end of a major amputation. The diabetic black toe with bounding pulses a few centimetres away is now well known to be a complication of infection, where septic vasculitis damages the digital vessels, which become occluded by septic thrombus. As they are end arteries, the result is gangrene of the area supplied by the affected arteries, as in this case.

The patient, a 74 year old retired builder with Type 2 diabetes of five years duration, presented as an emergency at Casualty with infection and necrosis of the second and third toes of the left foot (Stage 5 foot) (Figure 1.2a), and was referred to the Diabetic Foot Clinic. He had strong pedal pulses but absent vibration sense at the big toes. His X-ray was normal despite the full-thickness necrosis. He was admitted and treated with quadruple IV antibiotics, amoxicillin 500 mg tds, flucloxacillin 500 mg qds, metronidazole 500 mg tds and ceftazidime 1 g tds. His CRP was 155.2 mg/l and his WBC was 16.85×10^9/l, with neutrophils of 14.41×10^9/l. He had a double ray amputation within 24 hours of admission (Figure 1.2b). He grew *Staphylococcus aureus* from the wound swab and *Proteus mirabilis* and Group G *Streptococcus* from tissue samples taken in theatre. His antibiotics were focussed to amoxicillin, flucloxacillin and ceftazidime.

His recovery from the ray amputation was complicated by his development of frank painful haematuria. He had a past history of renal stones and had had a bladder stone removed in an open operation. His haemoglobin dropped from 11.3 g/dl to 8.2 g/dl and he underwent a blood transfusion. CT scan and ultrasound revealed a 5 mm calculus at the lower pole of the left kidney. MSU showed a heavy mixed growth and the patient was treated with ciprofloxacin 500 mg bd. His haematuria resolved and he was reviewed by the

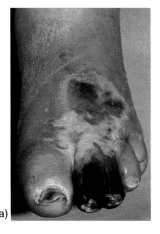
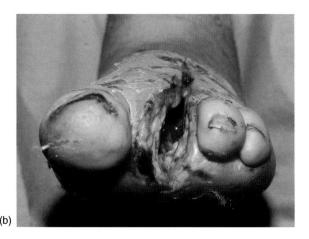

(a)   (b)

Figure 1.2   (a) Necrosis of the toes. (b) Double ray amputation.

urologists, who felt that no further treatment was necessary. His Type 2 diabetes was usually treated with oral hypoglycaemics but on admission, because of hyperglycaemia (20.5 mmol/l), he was treated with IV insulin sliding scale, which after two days was changed to a basal bolus insulin regime. Later on in the admission his foot wound grew *Enterococcus faecium* sensitive to vancomycin and teicoplanin. A PICC line was inserted into an antecubital vein, and he was discharged home on teicoplanin 400 mg daily IV and ciprofloxacin 500 mg bd orally. His foot healed after six weeks and the orthotists made him two pairs of shoes with cradled insoles. After healing of the foot, his diabetic therapy returned to metformin and glargine insulin at bedtime. He attended the Diabetic Foot Clinic regularly for nail care and removal of callus and his foot did not relapse.

Learning points

- Diabetic patients with Type 2 diabetes often have evidence of complications at the time of diagnosis because of glucose intolerance that may have been present for some years. Thus it is not surprising for this patient, who has a known history of diabetes for five years, and probably had glucose intolerance for some years before that, to have profound neuropathy.

- This patient had a typical polymicrobial infection of the diabetic foot, with *Staphylococcus aureus*, Group G *Streptococcus and Proteus mirabilis* isolated. The latter two organisms were isolated from operative tissue samples, thus illustrating the critical importance of sending operative tissue for culture. All three organisms in this polymicrobial culture were important and each needed appropriate antibiotic therapy.

- Many patients with Type 2 diabetes and foot infections will need insulin during the period of foot sepsis and subsequently during wound healing.

- Patients with Type 2 diabetes often have multi-system disease. Recovery from diabetic foot infections can be complicated by other illnesses, which need prompt attention or else they may compromise healing of the foot.

- Diabetic patients with urinary tract calculi are particularly prone to complications, especially infection.

Case 1.3 Neuropathic ulceration and infection lead to severe metabolic disturbance

When infection is not caught early and controlled well, then patients can become very ill. This poor lady went to see her general practitioner as soon as she detected an ulcer, but even so she developed severe foot problems.

The lady was 64 years of age and had had Type 1 diabetes for 25 years. She developed a small ulcer on the right first toe. It was her first foot ulcer. She visited her general practitioner, who prescribed flucloxacillin 500 mg qds. She had atrial fibrillation and was taking warfarin and digoxin. The next morning she felt unwell and was short of breath, and vomited on two occasions. Her family took her to Casualty. She had interdigital sepsis between the first and second toes with spreading cellulitis but good foot pulses. She had painless full thickness necrosis on the lateral aspect of the first toe with wet gangrene. She also had wet necrosis of the second toe, with infection extending up the tendon sheath, and wet gangrene of the medial aspect of the third toe. The plantar fat pads were necrotic in the base of the second and third toes (Stage 5 foot) (Figure 1.3a–d). She was in fast atrial fibrillation. Blood pressure was 60/30 mm Hg., CRP was 474 mg/l, WBC 23.82 $\times$ 10^9/l, with neutrophils 21.81 $\times$ 10^9/l, glucose 50.6 mmol/l, creatinine 152 μmol/l, sodium 129 mmol/l. She had evidence of ketoacidosis. The pH of arterial blood was 7.05 (normal values 7.35–7.45) and urine showed +++ ketones. Her INR was 7.22 (when anticoagulated we

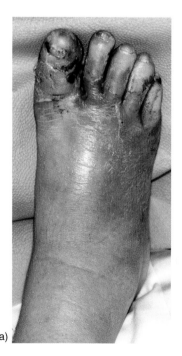

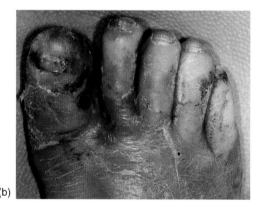

(a)   (b)

Figure 1.3 (a) Panoramic view of foot and lower leg. (b) Close-up of foot shows dorsal cellulitis.

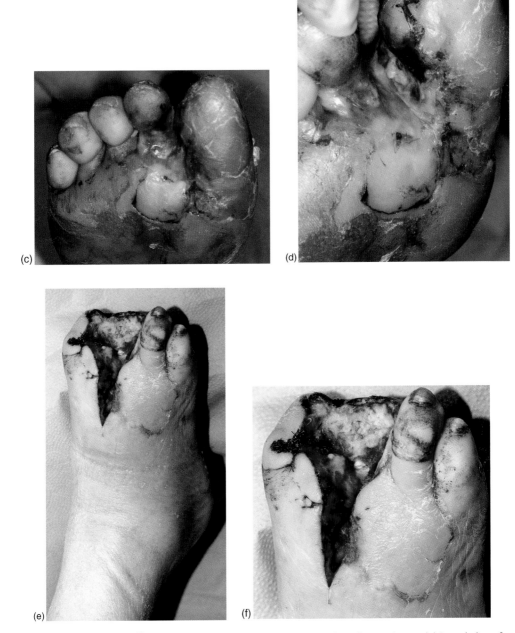

Figure 1.3 *(continued)* (c) Plantar view of foot. (d) Close-up view of necrotic toe. (e) Dorsal view of foot after surgery. (f) Close-up view of healing wound.

aim for INR around 3). A diagnosis was made of severe foot sepsis, diabetic ketoacidosis, cellulitis, fast atrial fibrillation and a deranged clotting mechanism secondary to her warfarin therapy and complicating sepsis.

She needed resuscitation in the Intensive Care Unit and was given amiodarone to control atrial fibrillation, IV insulin sliding scale and vitamin K and fresh frozen plasma. She was treated with IV amoxicillin 1 g tds, flucloxacillin 1 g qds, metronidazole 500 mg tds and ceftazidime 1 g tds. She underwent amputation of the right first toe, right second toe, and right third toe at the metatarsophalangeal joint (Figure 1.3e, f). The tissue cultures grew *Staphylococcus aureus* and Group B *Streptococcus* and antibiotics were narrowed down to amoxicillin and flucloxacillin. After the initial medical stabilisation followed by surgical debridement, she then had vacuum assisted wound closure (VAC) therapy. Warfarin had been restarted and ten days later the patient had bleeding from the dorsal part of the wound. The leg was elevated and a Kaltostat dressing applied. Her blood pressure was 95/60 mm Hg. Her INR was 2.8. She was transfused two pints of blood. She had no further untoward events, and was discharged with regular follow-up in the Diabetic Foot Clinic and the foot subsequently healed.

Learning points

- Diabetic patients with severe co-morbidities can destabilise and become very unwell in the presence of ulceration and infection. This lady's foot did not look severely infected at first presentation to the general practitioner. Over the subsequent 24 hours she developed necrosis and became unwell and on presentation to the hospital she was critically ill.

- The foot infection destabilised the patient's anticoagulant therapy and she presented with an INR of 7.22. It also destabilised her diabetes and she presented with a life-threatening ketoacidosis.

- Patients with severe diabetic foot infections and associated metabolic instability should be resuscitated and stabilised as quickly as possible and then taken to the operating theatre for surgical debridement. However, such resuscitation should be quickly achieved, as the patient with necrosis and spreading infection needs urgent surgical debridement. It may be said that a patient is too ill to go to theatre but in the presence of spreading infection and necrosis it might also be said that the patient is too ill *not* to go to theatre.

- VAC therapy is very useful in accelerating the healing of post-operative wounds in neuropathic feet.

- During her recovery the episode of bleeding was possibly associated with her anticoagulant therapy but the INR was in therapeutic range. Bleeding could have been exacerbated by VAC therapy. However, anticoagulation is a caution not a contraindication during VAC therapy.

- There was synergy between *Staphylococcus aureus* and Group B *Streptococcus*, which is an important pathogen to which diabetic patients are particularly susceptible. Both bacteria produce toxins.

Case 1.4   Cutting the mushrooms

A recent report from India demonstrated that a high proportion of diabetic foot injuries are sustained within the home, and this case fits into this category.

A 60 year old lady had Type 2 diabetes diagnosed 9 years previously. She had peripheral neuropathy and hypertension, and was taking metformin 850 mg bd. She sustained an injury when a dirty knife fell on the foot and pierced the dorsum of the foot. The injury occurred when she was in the kitchen, and the knife was a kitchen knife with which she had been chopping mushrooms. She presented at the Diabetic Foot Clinic, previously unknown to us, one day later, complaining of pain and swelling, and she had difficulty in weight bearing. Her temperature was 36.6 °C and her blood glucose was 18.4 mmol/l. Her pedal pulses were palpable. There was a small laceration between the first and second rays on the dorsum (Figure 1.4a) surrounded by swelling (Figure 1.4b). There was bruising to the base of the second and third toes and tenderness on palpation (Stage 3 foot). X-ray was normal. Ultrasound showed induration of the subcutaneous fat at the dorsum of the first webspace and plantar to the big toe. There was no hypervascularity and no collection, and flexor and extensor tendons were intact. It was presumed that the knife wound had tracked through the web space to the plantar side. The patient was admitted and was treated with IV antibiotics, amoxicillin 500 mg tds, flucloxacillin 500 mg qds, metronidazole 500 mg tds and ceftazidime 1 g tds because of the concern of possible deep infection. Her tetanus prophylaxis was not up to date so this was given. An ulcer swab from the laceration was negative. Her foot was reviewed twice a day, and for the first 24 hours she was put on IV insulin sliding scale. Diabetic control was subsequently obtained by changing the patient to a basal bolus regime of insulin. She made a full recovery, after which she went back to oral hypoglycaemic agents and was followed up in the Diabetic Foot Clinic.

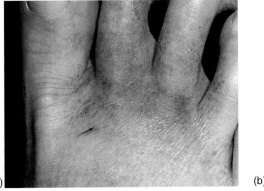
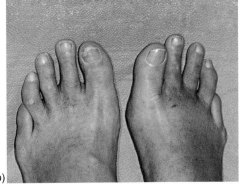

(a)   (b)

Figure 1.4   (a) Laceration from knife wound. (b) Swelling noted on lacerated foot compared with opposite foot.

Learning points

- Practitioners need to be careful about puncture wounds. Some of the worst cases of diabetic foot infections which we have seen began with a small and apparently innocuous wound.

- Practitioners should not be deceived by the seemingly trivial sign of a small puncture injury. Infection often is present at the base of the wound but then gradually takes hold.

- Speed of development of infection can be alarmingly rapid. Signs of infection after a penetrating injury only become apparent when the infective process has spread from the base of the puncture wound to the surrounding skin.

- Early presentation enabled this foot to be treated quickly and the risk of complicating infection to be averted.

- Pain is ominous in the neuropathic foot and should never be ignored.

- Puncture wounds often need admission to hospital as sepsis may be already apparent. Even when they are treated in the Diabetic Foot Clinic and not admitted, these patients should be reviewed every two to three days, despite the benign appearance of their foot.

- Many patients with severe infection will be apyrexial. Absence of fever – and even a normal white blood cell count – does not indicate that all is well and there is no infection.

- This lack of signs can make the patient even more difficult to manage, since a valuable sign of improvement is a decreasing temperature in a feverish patient.

Case 1.5   Infection leading to deformity

Although deformity usually leads to ulceration and then infection, occasionally infection can lead to tissue damage and then deformity.

This patient was 56 years old and had Type 2 diabetes for 5 years. She was obese and had a history of pulmonary emboli and was on warfarin therapy. She developed infection over the lateral aspect of the left foot with an ulcer probing to bone over the base of the fifth metatarsal (Figure 1.5a) (Stage 4 foot). She was admitted to hospital. She had a CRP of 54.6 mg/l and a WBC of 12.16×10^9/l with neutrophils of 9.24×10^9/l and was treated initially with amoxicillin 500 mg tds, flucloxacillin 500 mg qds, metronidazole 500 mg tds and ceftazidime 1 g tds. Deep wound swabs grew *Escherichia coli*, *Pseudomonas aeruginosa* and *Serratia marcescens*, all sensitive to piperacillin/tazobactam, to which she was changed, and her cellulitis resolved. However, she gradually developed an inversion deformity of the foot (Figure 1.5b) and was readmitted with recurrent sepsis. A swab grew *Enterobacter cloacae*, which was again treated with piperacillin/tazobactam. Her deformity has been accommodated in a total contact cast and her ulcer is healing. Surgery to correct the inversion deformity is under consideration, although the patient's past history of pulmonary emboli and obesity render her very high risk. She also has lymphoedema following her recurrent infection, and associated problems with healing an oedematous

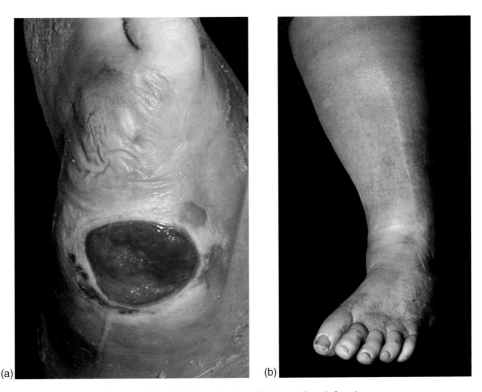

(a)   (b)

Figure 1.5   (a) Infected ulcer. (b) Inversion deformity.

limb are further reasons to avoid surgery. She has subsequently undergone successful reconstructive surgery of the foot. (Note added in proof)

Learning points

- Patients who have infections of the lateral foot often incur direct damage to the insertion of the peroneus brevis tendon to the lateral aspect of the base of the fifth metatarsal. Peroneus brevis is responsible for plantar flexion and eversion of the foot at the ankle. Damage to the insertion of the peroneus muscle leads to an inversion deformity.

- Ulceration and infection over the lateral aspect of the foot should be treated aggressively to prevent damage to the insertion of peroneus brevis.

- When the foot is debrided surgically for infection over the lateral aspect of the foot, care should be taken to preserve peroneus brevis function.

- Once this inversion deformity has developed the patient's foot should be accommodated in appropriate supportive footwear.

- This patient's initial foot cultures grew *Escherichia coli*, *Pseudomonas aeruginosa* and *Serratia marcescens*. These gram negative organisms are often regarded as insignificant in the diabetic foot. However, we believe that this is not correct. These bacteria can be definitely pathogenic in the diabetic foot, especially when they are in a pure growth or as part of a polymicrobial deep infection.

- Gram negative organisms should receive appropriate antibiotic therapy. Oral agents that are available to treat gram negatives are ciprofloxacin and trimethoprim. Parenteral agents include ceftazidime, aminoglycosides, meropenem, piperacillin/tazobactam, ticarcillin/clavulanate, tigecycline and ertapenem. It is crucial to obtain sensitivity patterns with gram negative organisms and not depend on empirical therapy alone.

Case 1.6 Neuropathic ulceration, sepsis, cardiac failure and more

This case was a lady with breast cancer, which was diagnosed during her admission for foot infection, and she also developed cardiac failure. Achieving healing of her foot was an urgent consideration so that she could commence chemotherapy for the cancer.

This 55 year old lady with Type 2 diabetes for 6 years presented with a necrotic ulcer of the right first toe, which was gangrenous at the base (Stage 5 foot). She also had a left-sided 10 cm labial abscess. She was admitted and treated with antibiotics comprising IV metronidazole 500 mg tds and vancomycin 1 g statim and then dosage as per serum levels and oral ciprofloxacin 500 mg bd. She was allergic to penicillin. A Group B streptococcus was grown from the labial abscess and the right toe necrotic ulcer. She underwent minor amputation of the first toe (Figure 1.6). However, post-operatively she had a pneumonia, which was treated with IV clarithromycin 500 mg bd. She was also put on insulin on a basal bolus regime. The patient also developed heart failure with pulmonary oedema, pulmonary hypertension and pleural effusions. An echocardiogram showed the left ventricle to be moderately dilated with normal left ventricular wall thickness, but left ventricular systolic function was reduced. She was treated with frusemide 80 mg orally, ramipril 10 mg orally, bisoprolol 1.25 mg orally and bendroflumethiazide 2.5 mg orally. She was also noted to have a lump in her breast with palpable axillary nodes. CT staging confirmed clinically locally advanced left breast cancer with involved axillary nodes. Every effort was made to control infection and heal the post-operative wound so that the patient could start chemotherapy.

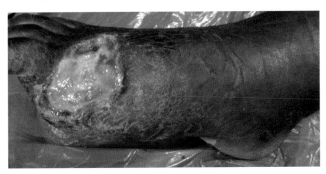

Figure 1.6 Postoperative healing wound.

Learning points

- This patient had Group B streptococcus from the labial abscess and the foot. This is increasingly recognised as an important pathogen in the diabetic patient.

- Diabetic patients with ulcers and infection may develop complications such as impaired cardiac function related to the infection. These need appropriate and accurate treatment to facilitate healing of the ulcer.

- This patient had significant complications, which impacted on the healing of the post-operative wound, particularly congestive cardiac failure. This needed urgent treatment to relieve the oedema and promote healing.

- It was also important to achieve healing of her post-operative wound as quickly as possible and control infection, so that the patient could start chemotherapy for her breast cancer.

Case 1.7   Infection in the neuropathic foot and Charcot foot

A useful technique for healing ulcers that have been surgically debrided following infection is vacuum assisted wound closure (VAC), which was used in the following case.

This was a 46 year old patient with Type 1 diabetes for 22 years who had peripheral neuropathy, autonomic neuropathy and proliferative retinopathy. He developed cellulitis over the dorsum of the right foot complicated by necrosis (Stage 5 foot). At his initial visit, when he presented with cellulitis, his foot swab grew Group B *Streptococcus* and he had a WBC of 14.87×10^9/l and a CRP of 157.6 mg/l, falling to 116.2 mg/l two days later. He was treated initially with IV amoxicillin 500 mg tds, flucloxacillin 500 mg qds, metronidazole 500 mg tds and ceftazidime 1 g tds, and underwent surgical debridement of the necrotic area (Figure 1.7a). Post-operatively this was treated with VAC therapy (Figure 1.7b). He was discharged on oral amoxicillin 500 mg tds, flucloxacillin 500 mg qds and metronidazole 400 mg tds. He was readmitted electively for a split skin graft to the previously debrided wound (Figure 1.7c).

However, after discharge he developed swelling of the right foot and an area of necrosis on the lateral right foot at the distal end of the previous skin graft. He underwent further surgical debridement of the right foot and further VAC pump therapy. Four weeks later it was noted at a Foot Clinic appointment that his right foot was swollen. Discharge from the wound had not increased, and there was no obvious cellulitis or fever. His WBC was normal. An X-ray (Figure 1.7d) showed lucency in the navicular and an MRI showed bony oedema of the tarsal bones in keeping with Charcot foot and a fracture of the navicular (Figure 1.7e). He was treated with an Aircast and the Charcot foot became non-active six months later and the wound healed.

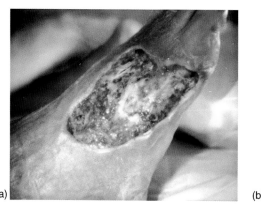
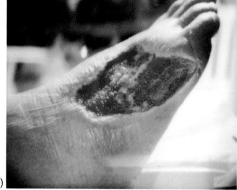

(a)   (b)

Figure 1.7   (a) Dorsal view of foot showing wound after debridement. (b) Dorsal wound after VAC therapy.

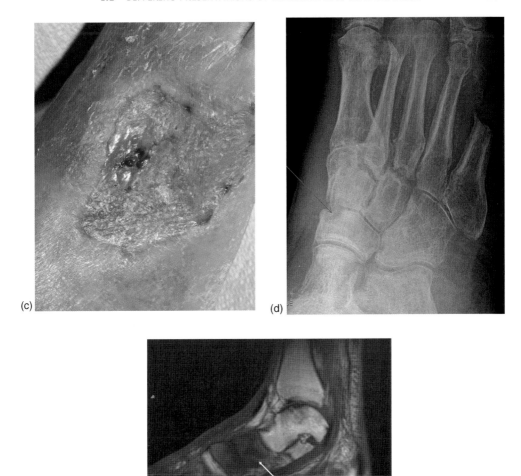

Figure 1.7 (*continued*)   (c) Skin graft. (d) X-ray shows lucency of navicular (arrow). (e) MRI (T1, sequence) showing oedema of tarsal bones and fracture of navicular (arrow).

Learning points

- When the patient returned with a swelling of the right foot, it was difficult to be sure clinically whether this was a relapse of infection or the onset of an acute Charcot foot. There was no raised WBC or fever but these are unreliable indicators of infection. However, imaging with X-ray and MRI demonstrated typical Charcot changes.

- When imaging with X-ray and MRI does not distinguish between osteomyelitis and Charcot, it is best to treat for both conditions.

- The trauma of undergoing surgical debridement may have precipitated his Charcot foot.

- He was treated in an Aircast instead of a total contact cast in view of his history of developing necrosis, because the Aircast could be removed for daily wound inspection.

- We often use the VAC therapy on large neuropathic wounds. This can speed up the formation of a granulating bed suitable for application of a skin graft, and we also use the VAC to speed healing of skin grafts. However, we wait for 24 hours after surgery before applying the VAC, and apply it with caution to patients who are on anticoagulants.

Case 1.8   Group A streptococcal infection

Group A streptococcal infection is rare in the diabetic foot but can cause extensive tissue damage.

This 74 year old patient with Type 2 diabetes for 15 years was bitten in Ghana by an insect on the left anterior leg. The leg became swollen, painful and cellulitic, and then developed multiple bullae, which were haemorrhagic, leading to areas of necrosis on the skin (Stage 5 foot) (Figure 1.8a, b). He took a plane back to the UK and came straight to King's Casualty. He was admitted. His CRP was 386.7 mg/l and creatinine 146 μmol/l with eGFR of 44 ml/min and his WBC was 14.5×10^9/l with neutrophils at 12.46×10^9/l. He had a fever of 38.7 °C. Malarial screen was negative. A deep wound swab grew Group A *Streptococcus*.

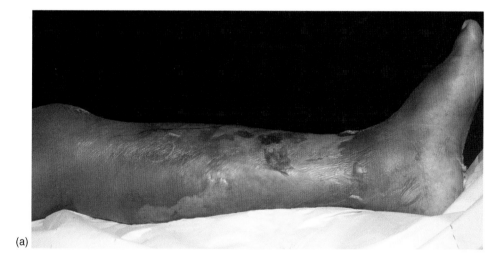

(a)

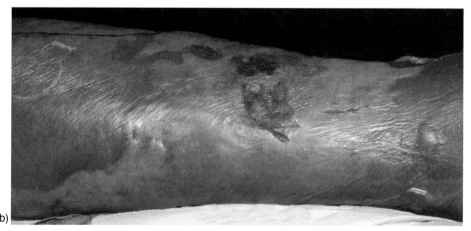

(b)

Figure 1.8   (a) View of the medial leg showing erythema, bullae and necrosis. (b) Close-up view of leg.

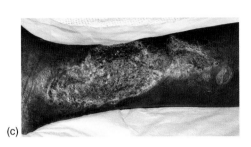
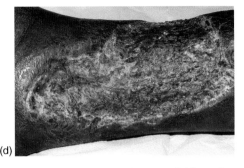

Figure 1.8 *(continued)*   (c) Debrided lateral leg with skin graft applied. (d) Close-up of skin graft.

The patient was initially treated with IV piperacillin/tazobactam 4.5 g tds and vanco-mycin 1 g statim and then dosage as per serum levels and then high dose IV benzylpenicillin 2.4 g qds when microbiology results were available. He was given sliding scale IV insulin. Areas of further necrosis developed and he underwent operative debridement and fasciotomy. His CRP dropped to 297 mg/l but returned to 395 mg/l with a WBC of 19.82×10^9/l with 17.35×10^9/l neutrophils. He needed two further debridements to achieve complete eradication of Group A *Streptococcus*, and a skin graft to achieve healing (Figure 1.8c, d). Over the subsequent six weeks his CRP fell to within normal range and his creatinine fell to 77 µmol/l.

Learning points

- Group A *Streptococcus* can cause severe infection in diabetic patients as well as non-diabetic patients. It is recognised by the widespread cellulitis, bulla formation, which is often haemorrhagic, and extensive necrosis involving skin, muscle and fascia.

- Aggressive IV antibiotic therapy and prompt surgical debridement are crucial to the successful management of these infections.

- The antibiotic of choice is penicillin, to which Group A *Streptococcus* is particularly susceptible and has not been found to be resistant.

- This patient underwent fasciotomy because of the excessive swelling associated with deep infection. Subsequently he underwent surgical debridement on two occasions to remove all necrotic tissue.

- In the Afro-Caribbean leg it can be difficult to assess the extent of necrosis.

Case 1.9 A gas leak

Many neuropathic patients present late with extensive tissue destruction and polymicrobial infection.

A 45 year old chef with poorly controlled Type 2 diabetes of 9 years' duration, retinopathy, nephropathy and autonomic and sensory neuropathy walked barefoot at home and trod on a tin tack. When he saw blood on the floor he realised that there was a problem and pulled the tack out with a pair of pliers and applied a sticking plaster. Two days later the puncture wound appeared to have healed. Five days later he developed a large blister on the dorsum of his foot and applied papaya ointment, a traditional remedy for wounds in the West Indies. The foot did not improve and gradually became very swollen so he attended Casualty, ten days after the original injury. The Diabetic Foot Clinic team was called down to Casualty to see him. He had a fever of 39.0 °C with rigors. The dorsalis pedis pulse could not be palpated, but the posterior tibial pulse was bounding. The foot was swollen with blistering and dark blebs on the dorsum, and when palpated there was crepitus and pus oozed from deep within the foot (Stage 5 foot) (Figure 1.9a). When a scalpel was inserted into the dorsum of the foot in a bedside procedure there was an audible hiss of escaping gas. The foot smelled terrible and the odour literally made the eyes sting.

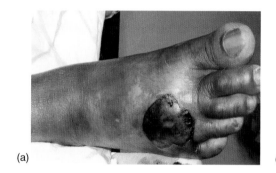
(a)

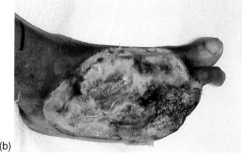
(b)

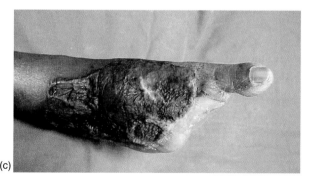
(c)

Figure 1.9 (a) Severe infection with bullae on dorsum of foot. (b) Post debridement. (c) Healed foot.

X-ray showed extensive gas within the soft tissue. Blood glucose was 27 mmol/l, CRP 279.6 mg/l and WBC 19.17×10^9/l with 16.30×10^9/l neutrophils.

Quadruple therapy with IV antibiotics of amoxicillin 500 mg tds, flucloxacillin 500 mg qds, metronidazole 500 mg tds and ceftazidime 1 g tds was commenced. He underwent an extensive debridement and amputation of third, fourth and fifth toes (Figure 1.9b) on the same day, and all debrided material was sent to the laboratory for microscopy and culture. He grew *Citrobacter koseri* sensitive to gentamicin, ciprofloxacin and ceftazidime, mixed anaerobes sensitive to metronidazole and MRSA sensitive to vancomycin from the debridings. In view of the culture of MRSA, the amoxicillin and flucloxacillin were stopped and vancomycin 1 g statim IV and then dosage according to serum levels was substituted and ciprofloxacin 500 mg bd orally added. He underwent further surgical debridement including amputation of the second toe. The wound was inspected twice daily. There was no further collection of gas, and the CRP fell steadily and his temperature remained down. After three weeks, during which time the wound was irrigated with Milton twice daily, a healthy bed of granulation tissue had been achieved and a split skin graft was applied, and the wound healed in one month (Figure 1.9c). He was followed up in the Diabetic Foot Clinic. He was very reluctant to wear bespoke shoes ("cripple boots", as he called them) but agreed to wear a pair of boots with a design based on trainer-style sports shoes, and he was given two pairs. He also needed protective footwear for his kitchen work and this was manufactured according to a sample of protective footwear from work that he brought to the clinic.

Learning points

- Puncture wounds may appear to be small and insignificant but they can inject micro-organisms deep into the foot and cause devastating infections.

- Patients should be advised not to use traditional remedies but to seek help from an experienced Diabetic Foot Clinic as early as possible.

- *Citrobacter* is a genus of gram negative coliform bacteria in the Enterobacteriaceae family, which can be found in the gut. It can be responsible for soft tissue infections in diabetic feet.

Case 1.10   Trouble on holiday: severe infection in a neuropathic foot

In Africa, extensive tissue loss is a feature of the diabetic foot. With the ease of modern travel, patients developing foot infections in Africa can readily present in other parts of the world.

A 62 year old African man, with Type 2 diabetes of 14 years' duration, presented to Casualty with a very swollen right foot with marked bulla formation and cellulitis (Stage 4 foot). He had noted swelling of the foot for a week and this had started whilst he was in Nigeria. His foot pulses were palpable. He had a pyrexia of 38.4 °C and a high WBC of 17.0×10^9/l, and his CRP was 200 mg/l. His blood glucose was 25.0 mmol/l. He was admitted to hospital, given IV amoxicillin 500 mg tds, flucloxacillin 500 mg qds, metronidazole 500 mg tds and ceftazidime 1 g tds and also given IV insulin sliding scale. He was taken to the operating theatre the same day and underwent radical surgical debridement to remove all of the infected tissue. He had necrotising fasciitis. Three toes and their adjoining rays were amputated and the remaining first and second toes were denuded of proximal dorsal skin as was most of the dorsum of the foot and the dorsal wound extended above the ankle (Figure 1.10a). However, the plantar skin was intact (Figure 1.10b). A specimen of this tissue grew *Proteus mirabilis* and *Escherichia coli*.

He was initially treated with quadruple antibiotic therapy, which was then focused to amoxicillin and ceftazidime, and he made a complete recovery. He was left with a considerable loss of tissue cover on the dorsum. A VAC pump was used to stimulate formation of a bed of granulation tissue (Figure 1.10c) after which it was successfully skin grafted (Figure 1.10d). Bespoke footwear was provided to prevent overloading of the remaining plantar surface. This area had good fibro-fatty padding and no plantar scarring.

He had an admission two years later for multiple abscesses and severe infection of the right upper arm, right forearm and right chest. X-ray showed subcutaneous gas and soft tissue swelling. MRI showed a large collection in the right arm within the anterior and posterior subcutaneous fat and extending through the biceps muscle belly. The collection also extended to the anterior chest wall deep to the pectoralis muscle and to the right lateral chest wall deep to and within the serratus muscles and around towards the back and extending across the axilla. There were pockets of gas. Two blood culture bottles grew a Group B streptococcus. CRP was 429.0 mg/l with WBC 29.32×10^9/l, and neutrophils 26.60×10^9/l. He had surgical debridement. Six months later he was admitted with a right sided lateral plantar ulcer and cellulitis, after presenting late with advanced infection. His CRP was 236.7 mg/l, WBC 14.48×10^9/l, neutrophils 11.42×10^9/l. He grew *Enterobacter cloacae* and was treated with amikacin 7.5 mg/kg/bd initially and then as per serum levels and meripenem 1 g tds IV.

The following year, he was admitted with a further foot infection and CRP of 236 mg/l, and a foot swab grew *Staphylococcus aureus*, Group B *Streptococcus* and *Enterobacter cloacae*, and blood cultures also grew Group B *Streptococcus*. He was again treated with amikacin 7.5mg/kg/bd initially and then as per serum levels and meripenem 1 g tds IV. He occasionally attends the Foot Clinic but frequently misses appointments, and despite his propensity to develop severe infections his approach to his feet is one of *belle indifference*.

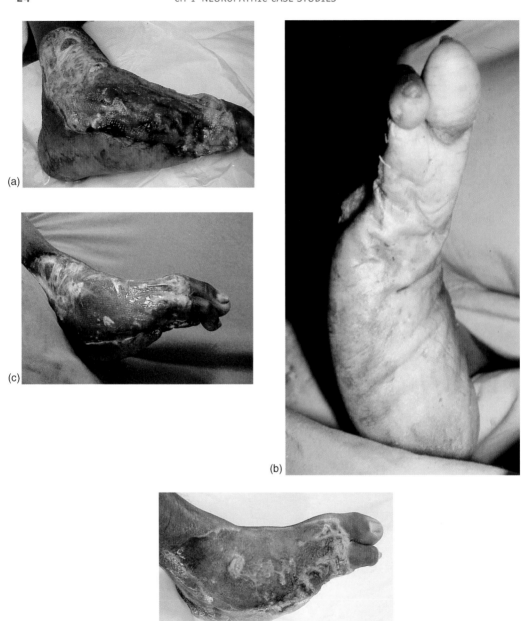

Figure 1.10 (a) Foot after surgical debridement. (b) Plantar skin. (c) Foot after treatment with VAC therapy. (d) Foot after successful skin graft.

Learning points

- Even a very small portal of entry, such as an insect bite, can lead to devastating infection, and patients from tropical countries may be particularly prone to develop these rapidly ascending infections.

- Necrotising fasciitis needs surgery without delay if the foot – and the patient's life – is to be saved.

- Wherever possible, the plantar tissues should be salvaged, as this will help to prevent further problems with neuropathic ulceration of the sole of the foot.

- The foot grew *Enterobacter cloacae*, a species of enterobacter that are enteric pathogens with limited sensitivities, being resistant to cephalosporins. Although laboratory testing may indicate sensitivity *in vitro* to the cephalosporins it is not advisable to treat with them, because enterobacter can induce chromosomal β-lactamases when challenged by a β-lactam antibiotic.

- Some surgeons believe that a transmetatarsal amputation should be performed if more than one ray needs to be removed, but it has always been King's policy to salvage as much as the foot as possible, since even if the foot is misshapen it can still function well with good foot care and footwear and orthotics.

- The VAC is a useful technique to obtain a good bed of granulation and to improve uptake of skin grafts.

Case 1.11   Denial leads to severe foot problems

Extensive tissue loss can also be a presentation of the neuropathic foot in the UK, especially when the patient has neglected his foot.

This 46 year old man had his Type 2 diabetes recently diagnosed when he had had a hospital admission with vomiting and fever. However, he refused any diabetic care or investigations. He was then admitted to hospital a year later with a large deep infection of the right foot extending over the lateral and dorsal aspects up to the ankle (Stage 5 foot). The second and fourth toes were already necrotic and the third toe had blue discoloration (Figure 1.11a–c). On admission there was a CRP of 187.5 mg/l. His creatinine was 51 μmol/l. WBC was 31.22×10^9/l, and neutrophils 27.67×10^9/l, indicating marked neutrophilia with a left shift in toxic granulation. X-ray of the right foot revealed osteopenia, but no injury was present. Glycated haemoglobin was 14.8%. Blood cultures were negative.

He was initially treated with quadruple IV antibiotics amoxicillin 500 mg tds, flucloxacillin 500 mg qds, metronidazole 500 mg tds and ceftazidime 1 g tds. Deep tissue swabs grew Group B *Streptococci* and *Staphylococcus aureus* and metronidazole and ceftazidime were stopped. He underwent extensive debridement of the foot, following which his CRP fell to 143.3 mg/l. Three days later a further surgical debridement was performed with amputation of the second, third and fourth toes. His wound was treated with VAC therapy (Figure 1.11d, e) and 18 days later he returned to theatre for further amputation of the first and fifth toes (Figure 1.11f) and his wound proceeded satisfactorily towards healing (Figure 1.11g).

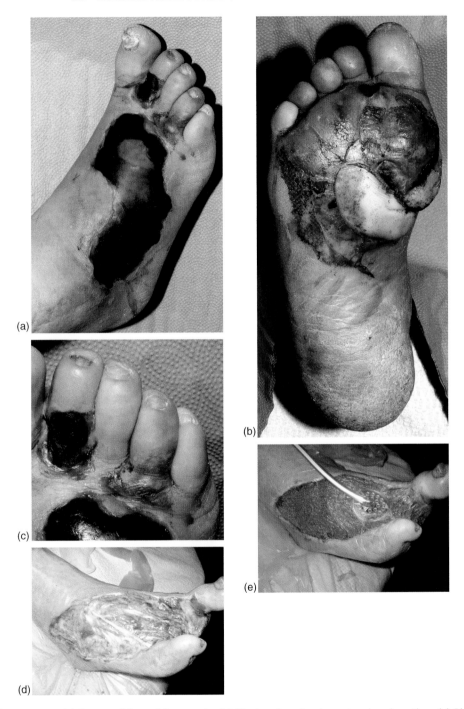

Figure 1.11 (a) Dorsum of foot with necrosis. (b) Plantar view showing extensive ulceration. (c) Blue discolouration of toes. (d, e) Post-operative wound before and after application of VAC therapy.

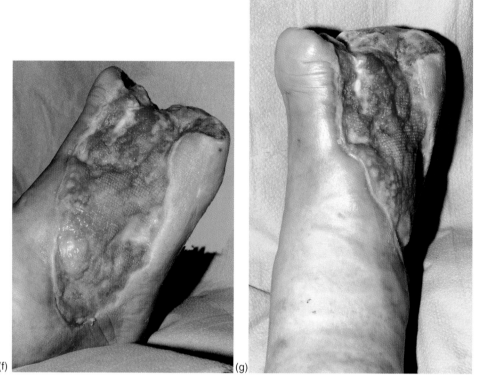

(f)   (g)

Figure 1.11 *(continued)*   (f) Amputation of all the toes. (g) Healing dorsal wound.

Learning points

- This gentleman had extensive tissue necrosis and he was considered for major amputation. However, he had a very good peripheral circulation and extensive surgical debridement with IV antibiotic therapy enabled the foot to be preserved.

- This needed very close working between diabetic and orthopaedic services.

- Very frequent observation of the foot is essential to determine when further surgery is required.

- When a patient does not accept that his diabetes is a problem or attends for appointments, then he becomes very prone to problems.

Case 1.12   The neuropathic foot and dermatological problems

Some patients with diabetic foot infections develop dermatological problems, as in the following case of DRESS syndrome.

This 60 year old patient with Type 2 diabetes for 5 years was admitted with severe left foot sepsis and necrosis (Stage 5 foot) (Figure 1.12a). His CRP was 203.9 mg/l, blood glucose 17.5 mmol/l, glycated haemoglobin 11.4%, WBC 20.35×10^9/l, with neutrophils 17.61×10^9/l. He was initially given quadruple IV antibiotics amoxicillin 500 mg tds, flucloxacillin 500 mg qds, metronidazole 500 mg tds and ceftazidime 1 g tds. He underwent incision and drainage and debridement. Extensive necrotic tissue was noted in both plantar and dorsal aspects and incision of necrotic ulcer edges was performed with curettage and debridement. A large communicating cavity was found on the mid-plantar aspect of the foot up to the toes extending up into the dorsal aspect of the foot and a large amount of pus was drained, and debridement of putrefied, necrotised tissue was performed. The fourth toe was non-viable, with no obvious blood supply and extensive, infective necrotic tissue throughout it, and the third toe was also non-viable. The second toe was noted to have necrotic tissue surrounding it.

The tissue cultures grew *Citrobacter koseri*, *Streptococcus milleri* and mixed anaerobes. After surgery the white count fell to 8.77×10^9/l. The patient subsequently developed a widespread oedematous erythematous maculopapular rash on his scalp, chest, upper back and right forearm (Figure 1.12b). The patient also had an eosinophilia and abnormal liver function tests, but ultrasound of the liver was normal. He was treated as DRESS syndrome (drug related eosinophilia with systemic symptoms) and given prednisolone 60 mg daily.

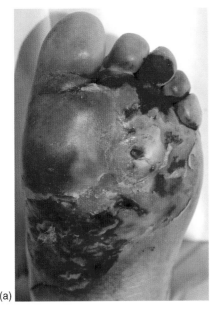

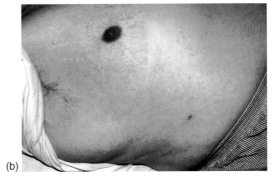

(a)   (b)

Figure 1.12   (a) Extensive cellulitis and necrosis. (b) Widespread rash.

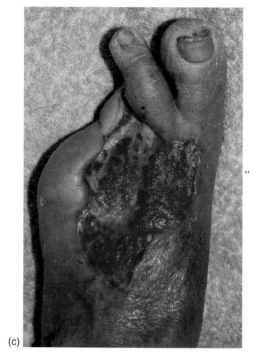

(c)

Figure 1.12 *(continued)*   (c) Healing foot.

Skin biopsy showed mild hyperkeratosis with minimal acanthosis, focal spongiosis and frequent apoptotic keratinocytes in the lower and, focally, in the upper layers of the epidermis. The superficial dermis contained a mild perivascular inflammatory cell infiltrate with scattered eosinophils. These features were in keeping with a drug reaction. The rash responded to prednisolone, which was gradually reduced in dosage and then stopped. The foot healed and he was followed up in the Diabetic Foot Clinic. Two months later, he had a relapse of his DRESS syndrome with an urticarial eruption over the left flank, which was again treated with a reducing dose of prednisolone. The foot continued to improve (Figure 1.12c).

Three months later, he had papules and nodules on the forearms and scalp as well as a demarcated linear papular urticated eruption on the right anterior cubital fossa. He was treated with Elocon (mometasone furoate) ointment to the inflamed areas of skin. After a further 3 months, the patient had a diffuse pruritic and erythematous rash on the chest and neck following treatment with metronidazole and was treated with chlorpheniramine. Finally, he developed thoracic shingles and was given acyclovir orally. He had residual post-herpetic neuralgia and was given dothiepin cream.

Learning points

- Diabetic patients with foot infections are exposed to many different antibiotics, which may provoke side effects including skin rashes.

- Dermatological drug reactions are self-limited diseases and therefore generally treatment is symptomatic. Prompt diagnosis and early withdrawal of all suspect drugs are the most important steps.

- Severe skin reactions include toxic epidermal necrolysis, Stevens-Johnson syndrome and DRESS syndrome, which stands for drug rash (or reaction) with eosinophilia and systemic symptoms.

- The symptoms of DRESS syndrome usually begin 1–8 weeks after exposure to the offending drug. Classic symptoms are rash, fever, lymphadenopathy and involvement of one or more internal organs. The rash is an erythematous skin eruption, often progressing to exfoliative dermatitis. It has a mortality rate of about 10%.

- DRESS syndrome responds to steroids, although it can relapse.

- This patient suffered a series of skin problems in which shared care with the dermatologists was crucial for accurate diagnosis and correct treatment.

- *Streptococcus milleri* is associated with pyogenic infection and abscess formation. Although often isolated in pure growth, it also found in polymicrobial infections.

Case 1.13   Diabetic patients with neuropathic feet may have a neuropathic bladder, which predisposes to urinary tract infections

The diabetic patient with neuropathy is prone to infection in other systems. Urinary tract infections are notable in diabetic patients with foot problems. These often emanate from a degree of neuropathy to the bladder: we have seen patients with distended bladders and concurrent foot problems, as in this case.

A 53 year old man with longstanding Type 1 diabetes for 48 years was admitted with ulceration and sepsis of the heel (Stage 4 foot). He was noted to have a distended abdomen and palpable bladder and urinary catheterisation drained 1500 ml of urine, which was cloudy and grew more than 100,000 organisms/ml of *Escherichia coli*, which was an ESBL (extended sensitivity β-lactamase) producer. The urinary tract infection responded to IV meropenem 1 g tds. A catheter was left in the bladder to drain completely for 12 hours. The patient then had urodynamic studies, which confirmed a neuropathic bladder, and this was treated by intermittent catheterization.

Learning points

- Patients presenting with neuropathic ulcer may have neuropathy affecting other systems of the body, and in particular the urinary tract.

- Symptoms are frequently masked by the neuropathy, so urinary retention should be actively sought since bladder distension is not painful in neuropathic patients.

- Bladder distension predisposes the patient to infection and a urinary culture should be obtained to detect the specific organisms so that appropriate antibiotic therapy can be prescribed.

- The *Escherichia coli* was an ESBL (extended sensitivity β-lactamase) producer. These organisms have developed resistance to extended-spectrum (third generation) cephalosporins (e.g. ceftazidime, cefotaxime and ceftriaxone) but not to carbapenems (e.g. meropenem or imipenem). ESBL enzymes are most commonly produced by two bacteria – *Escherichia coli* and *Klebsiella pneumoniae*. Another group of lactamases is AmpC β-lactamases, which are typically encoded on the chromosomes of many Gram negative bacteria including *Citrobacter*, *Serratia* and *Enterobacter* species, where expression is usually inducible. Thus, organisms considered susceptible by *in vitro* testing can become resistant during treatment with cephalosporins. These are gram negative organisms considered resistant to the cephalosporins and need treatment with the carbapenems.

Case 1.14   Prostatic obstruction

Although in a diabetic foot patient neuropathy may be the cause of a distended bladder, other aetiology such as prostatic enlargement should also be sought.

A 78 year old diabetic patient with Type 2 diabetes for 18 years was admitted with an infected ulcer on the right foot (Stage 4 foot) and had a surgical debridement by the orthopaedic surgeons. His serum creatinine quickly rose from 108 to 190 µmol/l, and then gradually fell to 106 µmol/l. The rise in creatinine was clearly associated with the episode of sepsis. At a routine measurement eight months later, the creatinine was normal, at 105 µmol/l, but three months after that it had risen to 264 µmol/l and the rising serum creatinine was initially assumed to be due to his diabetic nephropathy. After four more weeks it was 364 µmol/l. He was then admitted from the Diabetic Foot Clinic with a history of vomiting, fever and anorexia and a CRP of 177.3 mg/l. Although he had a small ulcer on the right foot there was no obvious focus of infection in the feet. Ultrasound of the kidneys and bladder showed both kidneys to be normal in size and shape. There was a bilateral hydronephrosis with an AP pelvic diameter of 2.7 cm on the left and 3.2 cm on the right. The bladder was of large volume and extended to the level of the umbilicus. There was a large residual volume after micturition of 1314 ml. Urine culture showed heavy mixed growth and he was treated with IV meropenem 500 mg bd. He had an enlarged prostate, which was clinically estimated to be 50 g. He did not want any active treatment, so a long term catheter was put in situ. His creatinine quickly fell to 130 µmol/l and did not rise again.

Learning points

- A raised serum creatinine in a diabetic foot patient may be related to diabetic nephropathy but there are other causes. Obstruction of the urinary tract should be investigated in all cases.

- The first rise of serum creatinine in this case history was related to infection in the foot. Although he had a foot ulcer at the time of the second rise in serum creatinine, it was not clinically infected, and indeed the second rise was related to the urinary tract infection and obstruction.

- Health care professionals working in Diabetic Foot Clinics have to be alive to the possibility of intercurrent illness in other systems in the body.

Case 1.15   Diabetic foot infection can masquerade as upper respiratory tract infection – always check the feet of diabetic patients

Although diabetic neuropathic patients with foot problems are prone to other infections including urinary infections, on certain occasions they do indeed have infection in their feet and a rise in inflammatory markers, which may mistakenly be attributed to infection elsewhere, including influenza.

This 40 year old patient with Type 2 diabetes for 6 years poorly controlled on metformin and glicazide first presented to Casualty complaining of flulike symptoms and cough. He was pyrexial and was a known asthmatic. He was treated with salbutamol nebulisers and sent home, with a diagnosis of a respiratory tract infection. His feet were not checked. The next day he came to the Diabetic Foot Clinic. He had infection of the left second toe with necrosis and cellulitis (Stage 5 foot) (Figure 1.15a). His foot pulses were palpable. He had a temperature of 38.6 °C. His CRP was 346 mg/l with a WBC of 9.62×10^9/l and neutrophils of 7.48×10^9/l (which is slightly raised).

He was admitted to hospital and initially treated with quadruple antibiotic therapy IV amoxicillin 500 mg tds, flucloxacillin 500 mg qds, metronidazole 500 mg tds and ceftazidime 1 g tds. Tissue grew *Staphylococcus aureus* and Group B *Streptococcus* and antibiotics were focussed down to amoxicillin and flucloxacillin. His foot X-ray was normal but that did not rule out osteomyelitis. His glycated haemoglobin on admission was 14%. He was given IV insulin sliding scale. He was treated with subcutaneous enoxaparin sodium as prophylaxis for deep vein thrombosis. In view of the necrosis he underwent amputation of the second toe (Figure 1.15b). Post-operatively he was treated with VAC therapy and made a good recovery, despite insisting on going home for Christmas earlier than the diabetic foot team thought was wise. He was switched to oral clarithromycin after he developed a maculopapular rash and the rash resolved. His foot healed.

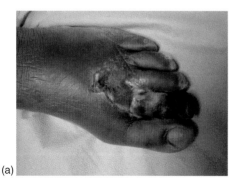
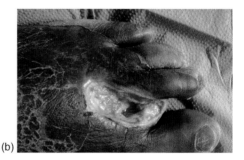

(a)   (b)

Figure 1.15   (a) Necrotic toe with spreading subcutaneous sloughing and cellulitis. (b) Amputation of second toe.

Learning points

- It should be mandatory to check the feet of any unwell diabetic patient.

- In this case, the patient had both a diabetic foot infection and a respiratory tract infection. When he presented on the second occasion with fever the respiratory tract infection diagnosed on the previous day could easily have been thought to be responsible for this, and it was only by checking the feet that his further foot infection came to light.

- All diabetic foot patients who undergo surgery and post-operative bed rest should receive venous thromboembolism prophylaxis.

- Osteomyelitis may not show up on X-ray for two weeks.

1.3   Co-Morbidities in addition to diabetes and neuropathy

Diabetic patients with neuropathy may have other co-morbidities, including microvascular and macrovascular complications. These patients may also have non-diabetic co-morbidities as well, which may further predispose them to ulceration and infection. These factors, in addition to peripheral neuropathy, may make them very vulnerable, as illustrated in the next series of patients, who demonstrated existing co-morbidities as they presented with their neuropathic feet. All these factors need active management to achieve resolution of infection and healing of ulceration.

Case 1.16   Diabetes, neuropathy and pancreatitis

This was a 51 year old man with Type 1 diabetes and an ongoing history of pancreatitis. He was admitted in diabetic ketoacidosis precipitated by acute pancreatitis and was treated in the Intensive Care Unit. He had clear evidence of neuropathy, with loss of sensation to mid-calf and absent vibration perception at the ankles bilaterally. He made a good recovery from his pancreatitis and was discharged, but eight weeks later he had a recurrence of his acute pancreatitis. During this admission a fissure on his left heel became infected, leading to cellulitis and osteomyelitis (Figure 1.16a). He was given IV piperacillin/tazobactam 4.5 g tds. Cultures from his heel grew *Staphylococcus aureus* and anaerobic *Streptococcus*. He underwent surgical debridement of the heel (Figure 1.16b) and two days after the operation he commenced VAC therapy. Seven days postoperatively he developed shortness of breath with right sided chest pain, and became hypoxic. On examination he had evidence of bilateral pleural effusions. Chest X-ray showed right sided basal consolidation. He underwent pulmonary angiography, which showed a filling defect in the right lower lobe subsegmental to the pulmonary artery, indicating a pulmonary embolus. His ECG did not show ischaemic changes and serum troponin I was less than 0.05 µg/l (lower limit of detection 0.05 µg/l), ruling out a myocardial infarction. His echocardiogram showed normal left ventricular systolic function. He was treated with therapeutic enoxaparin sodium. His heel improved on VAC therapy (Figure 1.16c), although he suddenly developed pain in his heel resulting from a pathological fracture of the calcaneum. This was treated with a non-weight-bearing cast in which a window was cut to observe the heel wound. Both fracture and wound eventually healed.

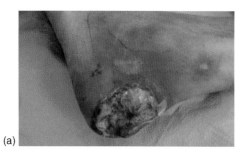
(a)

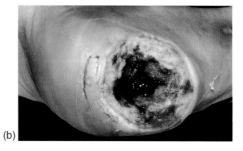
(b)

Figure 1.16   (a) Cellulitis and necrosis of the heel. (b) Post debridement.

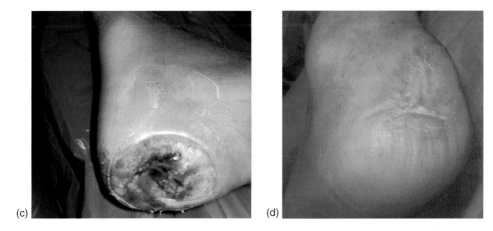

Figure 1.16   (*continued*) (c) Improvement on VAC therapy. (d) Healed wound.

Learning points

- Heel fissures are common problems on the diabetic foot and can act as portals of entry for infection. They should be treated early with debridement and emollients, to prevent ulceration.

- The calcaneal fracture was a pathological fracture related to osteomyelitis and underlying osteoporosis associated with his pancreatitis.

- Diabetic patients may not exhibit classical chest pain during episodes of ischaemia of the heart and the serum troponin is a measurement of cardiac tissue damage, which can be used in these circumstances to confirm or rule out a myocardial infarction.

- A serum troponin rise occurs in two situations. In ischaemic heart disease there is a rise in troponin because of the cardiac muscle damage from infarction secondary to thrombosis. Serum troponin also rises in septicaemia.

- It should be standard practice now for patients admitted to the hospital who are immobile to receive prophylactic anticoagulant therapy, as this patient did. Such therapy comprises a low molecular weight heparin such as enoxaparin sodium, which can be given subcutaneously once daily as long as the renal function is not significantly impaired, when heparin itself should be administered. Despite prophylactic anticoagulation in this case, the patient still developed a pulmonary embolus, which may have been related to his surgical debridement.

Case 1.17   Rheumatoid arthritis, neuropathy and an infected foot

Patients with diabetes and rheumatoid arthritis are very susceptible to ulceration and infection.

This 74 year old lady with Type 2 diabetes of 18 years' duration was referred to the Diabetic Foot Clinic by her general practitioner as an emergency. She lived with her 78 year old husband, who was in good health and drove her to the hospital in his own car. She had poorly controlled diabetes, despite taking maximum doses of oral hypoglycaemic agents, and a 40 years' history of rheumatoid arthritis, with severe deformity of feet and hands. This started when she was pregnant with her second child and had caused severe pain over the years, affecting her hands, wrists and elbows so that she could no longer play the piano, which caused her great sadness as she had been a talented amateur pianist. She also had problems with her ankles, knees and hips and she had undergone hip and knee replacements. She was taking methotrexate and prednisolone.

She had recently purchased a pair of "wide-fitting" shoes from a mail-order catalogue and had worn them around the house and on a visit to her daughter. "My wardrobe is full of almost-new shoes that I bought and can't wear because they make my feet hurt", she said. She had a VPT of 35 V and an ankle brachial pressure index of 1.00. She had severe hallux valgus of both feet. On the medial border of the right foot, directly over the prominent deformed forefoot there was a small ulcer with associated redness, warmth and swelling (Stage 4 foot). The base of the ulcer was yellow, soft and sloughy (Figure 1.17). She said that the ulcer itself was not painful but she had "deep pain" in both the feet whenever she walked. The ulcer did not probe to bone and an X-ray of the foot revealed severe erosions of the first metatarsophalangeal joint associated with rheumatoid arthritis, but no signs of infection in the bone. A diagnosis of soft tissue infection was made. She was admitted for IV antibiotics clarithromycin 500 mg bd and metronidazole 500 mg tds and oral ciprofloxacin 500 mg bd (she was allergic to penicillin), and the cellulitis resolved in five days and the foot healed after three weeks.

She was advised to use shoes that could accommodate the hallux valgus deformity, and agreed to this. Because of the severe deformity of the feet it was not possible to accommodate her in off-the-shelf, wide-fitting shoes, and bespoke boots were necessary. These had very deep and roomy toe boxes and deep cushioned insoles made of poron over a cradled insole to prevent her feet from rolling over into valgus and also supported her painful ankles. Heel counters were also fitted to increase her stability when walking, as she was very frail and unsteady and found it difficult to use crutches or sticks because they caused pain in her wrists and elbows. We asked the physiotherapists to review her and they visited her home and issued her with some helpful devices to make her life easier. She had no further foot problems but was seen regularly in the Diabetic Foot Clinic for nail care and regular review of the footwear. She was also followed in the Rheumatology Department. The King's Diabetic Foot Clinic ran a Friday morning satellite foot clinic for patients with rheumatoid arthritis, many of whom suffer from severe pain in the feet, and she attended this clinic, which was held concurrently with a rheumatology clinic, thus reducing the number of hospital appointments needed.

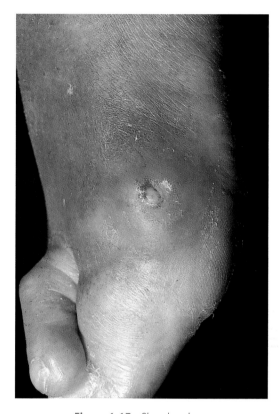

Figure 1.17   Sloughy ulcer.

Learning points

- Patients with rheumatoid arthritis may develop severe foot deformity. So long as there is no neuropathy they can often avoid ulceration because their feet are painful and they are careful to protect them, and if the feet are overloaded or the shoes are unsuitable the patient will be aware of the problem before it leads to ulceration. However, if they are also diabetic with peripheral neuropathy, as in the case of this lady, then foot ulceration is common. We have also seen cases of rheumatoid nodules of the feet that break down.

- Drugs used to treat rheumatoid arthritis predispose patients to infections, and rheumatoid patients who also have concurrent diabetes should be regarded as high risk patients.

- Diabetic foot patients should not purchase mail-order footwear without receiving advice from the Diabetic Foot Clinic, who should also check any shoes before the patient wears them.

1.4   Deformity, ulceration and infection treated by surgical debridement and reconstruction

Infections in the neuropathic foot often complicate ulcers that are associated with deformity. Long term outcomes improve if deformity can be corrected. In certain cases this correction can be carried out at the time of surgical debridement for an infection. We now describe four cases where reconstruction was successfully carried out at the time of their initial debridement. These patients were seen in the joint Orthopaedic/Diabetic Foot Clinic at King's, and we wish to pay special tribute to Mr. Venu Kavarthapu, Consultant Orthopaedic Surgeon, who carried out the reconstructions. All patients were followed up in the Diabetic Foot Clinic.

Case 1.18   Forefoot reconstruction can solve the problem of recurrent ulceration and sepsis associated with deformity

---

This was a 50 year old man with Type 2 diabetes for 10 years. Complications included maculopathy, peripheral neuropathy and hypertension. He had had previous amputations of the third and fifth toes. He developed a chronic ulcer under the second metatarsal head of the right foot, which was complicated by osteomyelitis. He was admitted as an emergency. He had a CRP of 70.9 mg/l and a WBC of 9.92×10^9/l with neutrophils 7.56×10^9/l (slightly raised). Although there was considerable cellulitis, no micro-organisms were grown. X-ray showed dislocation of the second metatarsophalangeal joint (Figure 1.18a). On MRI the second metatarsal showed abnormal signal on T1 and post-contrast extending through most of the metatarsal (Figure 1.18b). This was in keeping with osteomyelitis affecting almost all of the second metatarsal. The third metatarsal head showed abnormal signal on coronal section, again consistent with osteomyelitis (Figure 1.18c). All of these marrow changes appeared contiguous with extensive soft tissue change which extended up to the plantar ulcer.

The patient was treated with amoxicillin 500 mg tds, flucloxacillin 500 mg qds, metronidazole 500 mg tds and ceftazidime 1 g tds IV antibiotics, underwent right second and third metatarsal exploration and had excision arthroplasty and internal fixation with a wire in the second toe (Figure 1.18d). He was discharged home on ceftriaxone 1 g IM daily and metronidazole 400 mg tds orally. The wire was removed after 4 weeks, the ulcer healed quickly and the foot did not relapse in the subsequent year.

Learning points

- Patients with persistent ulcer secondary to deformity should be assessed to determine whether the deformity can be corrected surgically.

- Patients presenting with infection secondary to ulceration can be treated with IV antibiotics, surgical debridement to remove infected tissue and formal reconstructive surgery to correct deformity.

- Forefoot reconstruction techniques can be very successful in correcting digital deformities.

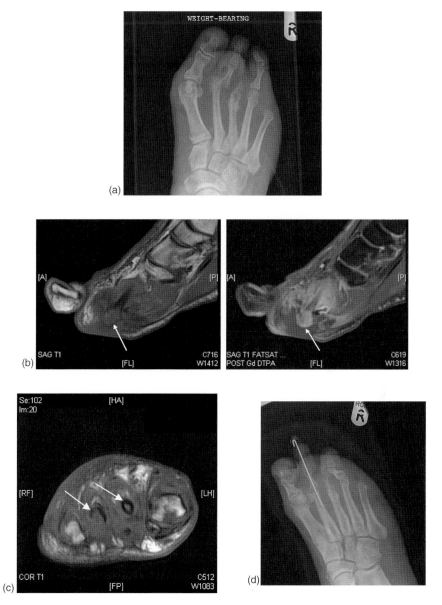

Figure 1.18 (a) X-ray shows dislocation of second metatarsophalangeal joint. (b) MRI sagittal sections of T1 and post gadolinium sequences showing oedema of second metatarsal head and shaft (arrow). (c) MRI coronal section showing oedema of second and third metatarsal heads (arrows). (d) X-ray following surgical procedure showing in situ wire in the second ray.

Case 1.19   The orthopaedic surgeon is a key member of the diabetic foot team

This 70 year old man had Type 1 diabetes for 40 years. His control was good with glycated haemoglobin of 7%. This patient first came to the Diabetic Foot Clinic 21 years previously presenting with ulceration of the left foot and also a left Charcot foot. His foot healed with podiatric debridement, antibiotics and an extended stay in hospital for bed rest. However, over the next 20 years he had many episodes of plantar ulceration. Despite receiving prolonged pressure relieving orthotics in the Diabetic Foot Clinic, the plantar ulcer did not heal. He was admitted as an emergency with infection of a plantar ulcer under the second metatarsal head. He had a fixed claw deformity, a stiff first metatarsophalangeal joint and a non-reducible chronically dislocated second metatarsophalangeal joint. The ulcer probed only to the soft tissues. X-ray showed, in the first and second metatarsophalangeal joint, loss of joint space, sclerosis and subchondral cysts. There was subluxation of the second metatarsophalangeal joint (Figure 1.19). He had a CRP of 38.2 mg/l and a WBC of 6.71×10^9/l, of which neutrophils were 4.91×10^9/l. He was treated with IV vancomycin 1 g statim and then dosage as per serum levels, metronidazole 500 mg tds and ceftazidime 1 g tds (he was allergic to penicillin). *Staphylococcus aureus* was grown from the foot ulcer swab.

He underwent surgical debridement and dorsal wedge shortening with Weil's osteotomy and proximal hemi-phalangectomy of the second toe of the left foot to correct the

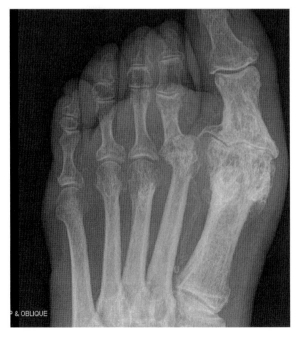

Figure 1.19   Foot X-ray showing subluxation of the second metatarsophalangeal joint and degenerative changes at the first metatarsophalangeal joint.

deformity that had predisposed him to recurrent ulceration. He was discharged on ceftriaxone 1 g IM daily and metronidazole 400 mg tds orally. His ulcer healed and his deformity was corrected.

Learning points

- Neuropathic patients with long term ulceration and recurrence should be assessed for any associated deformity that has been responsible for the ulceration.

- Where possible, these deformities should be corrected by the orthopaedic surgeon.

- When patients present with both infected ulceration and deformity it is now possible to perform surgical debridement and correction of deformity in the same operation. However, it is important that the infection has been investigated and the appropriate antibiotics administered intravenously to eradicate the infecting organisms.

Case 1.20 Very rapid deterioration of a patient with diabetic foot infection

This patient was 60 years old and had Type 2 diabetes for 24 years. He had had laser therapy for proliferative retinopathy. He attended with ulceration under the left first metatarsal head associated with mild cellulitis. His temperature at presentation to the Diabetic Foot Clinic was 37.2 °C. Over the subsequent 2 hours his cellulitis spread and he became very unwell. He vomited, and became faint and hypotensive. His WBC was $25.08 \times 10^9/l$ with a marked neutrophilia and CRP was 127 mg/l. Serum creatinine was normal at 117 μmol/l. He was started on quadruple IV antibiotics amoxicillin 500 mg tds, flucloxacillin 500 mg qds, metronidazole 500 mg tds and ceftazidime 1 g tds IV. His CRP was 178 mg/l on admission to the ward and next day rose to 264 mg/l. Blood cultures grew Group A *Streptococcus*, which was also isolated from his foot ulcer deep wound swab. He developed severe pain in his left groin and ultrasound showed multiple enlarged lymph nodes measuring up to 1.7 cm in short axis diameter. On the third day CRP had fallen slightly to 236 mg/l and white count was $18.57 \times 10^9/l$. Both parameters gradually fell over the following week and his cellulitis resolved. He was followed up in the Diabetic Foot Clinic, and the ulcer healed.

However, he had recurrent foot ulceration over the first metatarsophalangeal joint. Each episode was associated with cellulitis and he was very quickly treated with amoxicillin and flucloxacillin orally. He had one further admission with cellulitis and a CRP of 86 mg/l and slightly raised white count of $11.45 \times 10^9/l$ with $9.18 \times 10^9/l$ neutrophils. He was again treated with quadruple IV antibiotics as above. A deep wound swab grew *Staphylococcus aureus* and his antibiotics were focussed to flucloxacillin. It had not been possible to prevent recurrent ulceration with conservative therapy. X-ray showed a severe hallux valgus deformity with previous amputation of the second toe (Figure 1.20a). He underwent surgical debridement and correction of his left forefoot deformity with metatarsal osteotomy and fusion of the first metatarsophalangeal joint. In the anaesthetic recovery room, he collapsed and vomited and was treated for a possible aspiration pneumonia with meropenem 1 g tds IV. A postoperative chest X-ray was normal and foot X-ray showed internal fixation of the first metatarsal and proximal phalanx of the great toe as well as of the second and third metatarsal heads (Figure 1.20b). He has had no further episodes of ulceration over the subsequent year.

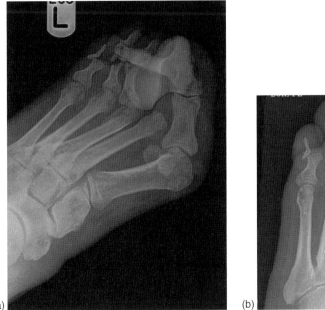
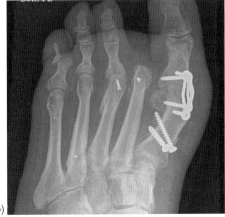

(a)   (b)

Figure 1.20   (a) Severe hallux valgus deformity with previous amputation of the second toe. (b) Internal fixation of the first metatarsal and proximal phalanx of the great toe as well as of the second and third metatarsal heads.

Learning points

- Diabetic patients with foot infection can become very unwell very quickly.

- Group A streptococcus can cause severe systemic symptoms.

- Pain in the groin from lymphadenopathy can be acute and can be indicative of a serious foot infection.

- The CRP usually reflects inflammatory events from the previous day.

- Recurrent foot ulceration associated with hallux valgus deformity should be addressed by correction of the underlying deformity.

Case 1.21 Indolent neuropathic ulceration

This patient was 48 years old with Type 1 diabetes for 33 years. She had a chronic non-healing ulcer on the plantar aspect of the right second metatarsophalangeal joint for 12 months despite cast therapy. She had a child and was very reluctant to undergo any treatment requiring hospital admission. However, she developed a foot infection with cellulitis and was admitted as an emergency for IV antibiotic therapy while her parents cared for her child. She was given antibiotics comprising IV vancomycin 1 g statim and then dosage as per serum levels, ceftazidime 1 g tds and metronidazole 500 mg tds as she was allergic to penicillin. She had a CRP of 73.7 mg/l and WBC of 10.52×10^9/l of which 8.32×10^9/l were neutrophils. Most previous wound swabs were negative, but one had shown MRSA. The cellulitis improved but her X-ray showed osteomyelitis of the second metatarsal head (Figure 1.21a). She underwent excision arthroplasty of the second metatarsophalangeal joint and Weil's osteotomy and proximal interphalangeal joint fusion of the fifth toe (Figure 1.21b, c). The alignment of the toes was satisfactory.

She was discharged with a CRP of 5.7 mg/l and a normal WBC, on teicoplanin 400 mg IM daily, and the ulcer healed after six weeks.

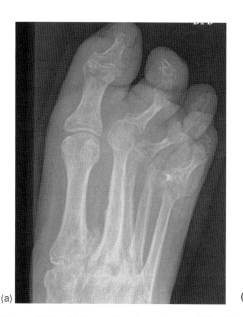

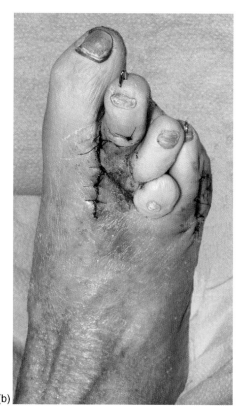

(a)   (b)

Figure 1.21 (a) X-ray showing osteomyelitis of the second metatarsal head. (b) Dorsal view of the postoperative foot.

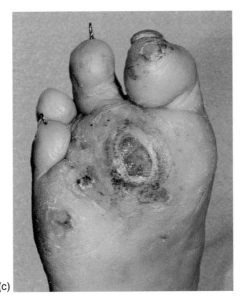

(c)

Figure 1.21 *(continued)* (c) Plantar view of the postoperative foot.

Learning points

- Long standing Type 1 patients with chronic recurrent foot ulceration often develop infection. Most episodes can be managed as an outpatient within the Diabetic Foot Clinic.

- Recurrent episodes of ulceration and infection can lead to chronic osteomyelitis and destruction of underlying bone and joint, which is best treated by excision arthroplasty.

- This lady avoided hospital admission for many years, but when an episode of ulceration was associated with severe sepsis necessitating hospital admission and IV antibiotics she was then able to accept surgery.

1.5 Patients with neuropathic feet in whom psychological factors have impacted on their management

Concurrent psychological problems can lead to enormous barriers to care. The six patients described below cover a wide variety of mental health problems, personality disorders and inability to accept advice and treatment. Some patients have incorrect beliefs about how neuropathic ulcers develop and do not understand the association between neglected callus and subsequent ulceration. They need careful education. Some unfortunate patients actually cause their own ulcers, and even prevent them from healing. It is difficult to understand the motivation of these patients. Confrontation is not helpful: they will move away to another hospital where their psychological problems are not known. We have seen a small cluster of these patients: they are almost all young women. A previous history of eating disorders or brittle diabetes is often found, and several of our patients have been health care professionals.

Case 1.22   Neuropathic ulceration and psychiatric disease

This 65 year old man with Type 2 diabetes for 12 years and a history of paranoid schizophrenia attended the Diabetic Foot Clinic over many years. He developed ulceration and swelling over the left first toe (Figure 1.22a). On attending the Diabetic Foot Clinic for a routine appointment he was found to have deteriorated and now had osteomyelitis of his left first toe (Figure 1.22b), localised collection of pus, fever and CRP of 150.6 mg/l. He was advised that he needed hospital admission and first toe amputation but refused this. His foot swab grew *Pseudomonas* and he was treated with ciprofloxacin 500 mg bd as an outpatient. During this period he was attending his GP practice from Monday to Friday for daily dressing change and being attended by the district nurses at the weekends.

He returned after two weeks, during which time his foot deteriorated (Figure 1.22c). His temperature was 38.9 °C. He finally agreed to be admitted to hospital. On the ward, he was treated with piperacillin–tazobactam 4.5g tds. Blood cultures on admission demonstrated MRSA bacteraemia. Vancomycin IV 1 g statim and then dosage as per serum levels was started and the piperacillin–tazobactam was stopped. The patient was isolated according to the hospital's MRSA infection control policy. Previous specimens from the Diabetic Foot Clinic identified the patient to be MRSA negative. He continued to refuse amputation. The cellulitis settled after four weeks of IV antibiotic therapy He refused any surgical intervention to his left first toe. His CRP had fallen to 83.8 mg/l on discharge and he was followed up in the Diabetic Foot Clinic. He was given fusidic acid 500 mg tds and doxycycline 100 mg daily. Foot X-rays showed evidence of resolving osteomyelitis (Figure 1.22d) and the ulcer eventually healed (Figure 1.22e). The patient continues to attend the Diabetic Foot Clinic.

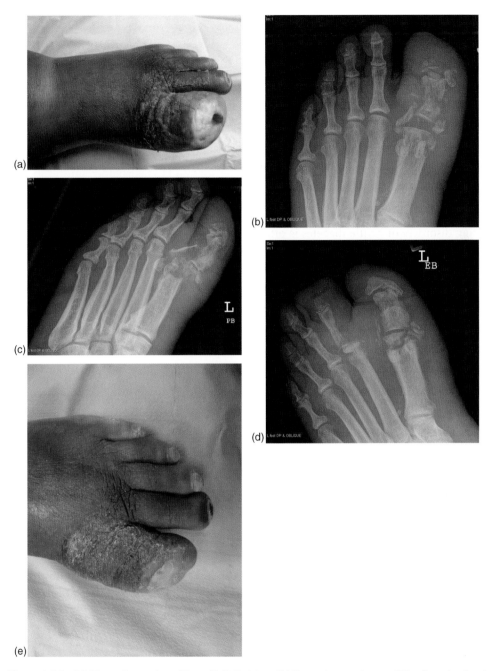

Figure 1.22 (a) Ulceration and swelling of left first toe. (b) X-ray shows osteomyelitis of proximal and distal phalanges of the left first toe. (c) X-ray shows worsening osteomyelitis. (d) X-ray showing reformation of proximal phalanx. (e) Healed ulcer.

Learning points

- Patients with mental health problems pose a great challenge and the Diabetic Foot Clinic is the ideal forum to follow them. It is their safe haven where they have continuity of care and often come to trust the personnel within it.

- It may not be possible to achieve all our goals and it may be necessary to compromise.

- This patient's ulcer eventually healed despite severe underlying bone destruction. Osteomyelitis can resolve on conservative treatment.

- It is always important to culture diabetic foot lesions and to take blood cultures so as to detect infecting organisms and bacteraemias including MRSA infections.

- Patients with MRSA infections should be isolated.

Case 1.23 In-growing toenail

A 59 year old man with Type 2 diabetes of 8 years' duration was referred to the Diabetic Foot Clinic by his general practitioner, when he visited him complaining of pain and throbbing in the right hallux, which was keeping him awake at night. His VPT was 15 V and pedal pulses were palpable. He lived alone following the death of his wife. The diabetes was well controlled with a glycated haemoglobin of 6%. He had never received foot care and had always cut his own nails. On examination the right foot was swollen, the medial nail sulcus of the right hallux was red and puffy (Figure 1.23) and pus was discharging from the medial sulcus. A diagnosis of onychocryptosis (in-growing toenail) was made. The medial sulcus was probed by the podiatrist and a splinter of nail that had penetrated the flesh was found and removed and the edge of the nail plate was smoothed with a Black's file so that it did not press upon the swollen sulcus. A dry dressing was applied. A swab was sent for culture, and oral amoxicillin 500 mg tds and flucloxacillin 500 mg qds were prescribed. Two days later the results of culture were received and checked against the patient's records to ensure that the antibiotics were appropriate. *Staphylococcus aureus* was grown, and the amoxicillin was discontinued. The foot healed in two weeks.

At his follow-up appointment, the patient was advised to cut his nails straight across and to ensure that he never tried to cut out the corner of the nail or left a splinter of nail behind

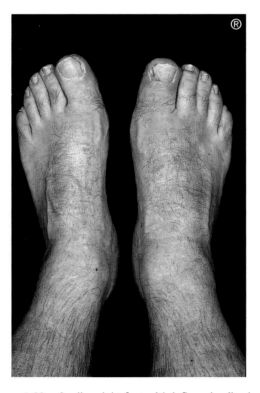

Figure 1.23 Swollen right foot with inflamed nail sulcus.

that might be forced into the flesh as the nail grew forward. He was advised to return to the Foot Clinic if any future problems arose and did not come back for ten years.

Unfortunately, his diabetes control had deteriorated, and he had developed complications. Initially the community podiatry service saw him and cut his nails and reduced callosities on the plantar surface of both feet. He developed a plantar ulcer on his left first metatarsal head; he was referred back to the Diabetic Foot Clinic by his community podiatrist, who was doing a training rotation working one day a week for three months at King's. She saw him at King's with the multidisciplinary team to ensure continuity of care. The foot was X-rayed: there were no signs of osteomyelitis. A swab was sent to the laboratory for culture: it grew *Staphylococcus aureus* and *Streptococcus* Group G and amoxicillin 500 mg tds and flucloxacillin 500 mg qds were again prescribed. The ulcer was debrided of callus. The orthotist made casts of both feet with a view to manufacturing bespoke shoes with cradled insoles. The ulcer healed in nine weeks and the patient continued to attend the Diabetic Foot Clinic every month and to see the Community podiatrist between these appointments. He lived alone, and gradually became unkempt in appearance and began to arrive late for appointments and sometimes to miss them. He also became very reluctant to wait to be seen if it was not possible for him to come into the clinic immediately. He arrived at the Foot Clinic one day wearing his bedroom slippers, saying that he had lost his bespoke shoes, but on the next visit he had found them again. On another occasion he wore unmatched shoes from two differently coloured pairs. He had no relatives or close friends to help him and was socially isolated. The general practitioner talked to him about his home situation: the patient was very reluctant to give up his home and move into sheltered accommodation, or to pay for a home help. He developed chronic neuropathic ulcers and the district nurses called daily to clean and dress his feet, but often he was not at home when they called. Close contact was maintained between the district nurses, the Foot Clinic, the community podiatry service and the GP practice, so that regular checks could be made on the patient's condition. He did not bathe regularly, and often did not take his medication regularly. Over the last two years of his life he had seven hospital admissions when his feet became infected. Use of a total contact cast to heal the ulcers was considered but it was felt that the risk of him not attending for review and developing devastating infection within the cast was too great for it to be risked. Eventually he failed to attend an appointment at the Foot Clinic, who notified the district nurses. They called at the house and could not gain entrance but spoke to a neighbour who was concerned because she had not seen the patient for two days. The police were asked to help. When they entered the house they found that the patient was dead. There was a coroner's inquest: the post-mortem revealed that he had died of a myocardial infarction.

Learning points

- Patients without significant neuropathy or peripheral vascular disease who can see their feet clearly are usually capable of self-care.

- All people with diabetes should be taught the principles of good nail care.

- If onychocryptosis does not settle and becomes a chronic problem then partial nail avulsion with phenolysation of the nail bed is an effective treatment, but is contra-indicated in patients with peripheral vascular disease.

- Nail conditions can lead to severe problems in the complicated diabetic foot and patients should receive expert help within a short time.

- Sometimes the home situation is not ideal and patients are unable to look after their feet well. In these circumstances, health care professionals have to make the best of the situation and endeavour to prevent catastrophes by offering frequent appointments and regular review. Home visits from the district nursing team are very useful.

Case 1.24 A patient's belief that podiatry caused a diabetic foot ulcer

A 58 year old woman with Type 1 diabetes of 38 years' duration was warned by her general practitioner that she should wear "sensible shoes" when she visited him and showed him a large area of callus on the plantar surface of her foot (Figure 1.24). He also wrote a referral letter to the Diabetic Foot Clinic asking if they could provide footwear, and she was seen later that week. She had palpable foot pulses and a VPT of 40 V. When the podiatrist debrided away the plantar callus a large blister was revealed. The patient became very upset, saying that the podiatrist had cut her foot and "caused an ulcer" and it was only after she talked to the diabetologist and the nurse that she understood that the problem had been present beneath the callus and that callus removal had only exposed the ulcer and not caused it. Dressings were applied and the patient was asked to rest and to return to the Foot Clinic in seven days' time, when the blister had healed. Bespoke shoes with cradled insoles were provided, and she remained ulcer free and attended the Foot Clinic regularly for callus removal and nail care.

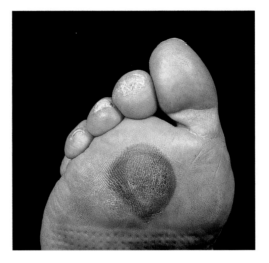

Figure 1.24 Callus with bulla.

Learning points

- Before callus or ulcers are debrided an explanation should be given to the patient as to the reasons for the debridement and the likelihood that an ulcer may be present beneath the callus.

- If patients become upset then a uniform response should be given by all the team members.

Case 1.25   Self-inflicted injuries

A 33 year old woman with poorly controlled Type 1 diabetes of 25 years' duration, proliferative retinopathy treated with laser, autonomic neuropathy and severe peripheral sensory neuropathy picked at her toenails instead of cutting them. She also had a habit of pulling pieces of loose skin off her heels, which were very dry. She was first seen in the Diabetic Foot Clinic when she first attended the Diabetic Department at King's at the age of 30 years. She was married with one small son. She had been referred to King's for "brittle diabetes", having had many episodes of ketosis requiring hospital admission and also complained of hypoglycaemia of sudden onset, of which she had no warning, which made it impossible for her to drive a car. When the condition of her toenails was noted she was offered treatment in the Diabetic Foot Clinic but refused to attend. She was referred to the Diabetic Foot Clinic again three years later, after attending the Diabetic Clinic for annual review. A random capillary glucose was unusually high, at 22 mmol/l and removal of her footwear revealed a hot swollen right foot with a blueish hallux. She said that two days before she had pulled off a loose piece of skin and the toe had bled but had not hurt. She was very reluctant to accept that admission was necessary, but telephoned her husband who came to the hospital and persuaded her to come in. Intravenous antibiotics were administered: however, the hallux gradually became black and necrotic and was amputated by the orthopaedic surgeon (Figure 1.25a). She was anxious to go home as soon as possible as she wanted to be with her family. Her small son became very upset every time his mother

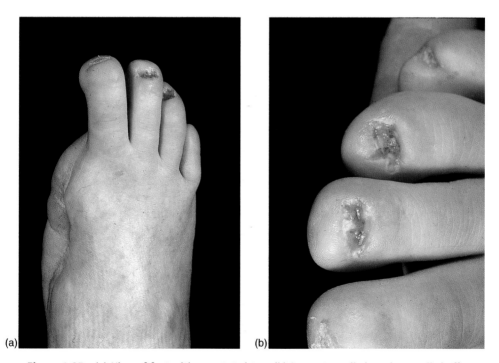

(a)   (b)

Figure 1.25   (a) View of foot with amputated toe. (b) Lesser toenails have been pulled off.

was admitted. She went home after two weeks in hospital. She was given an appointment the following week to come to the Foot Clinic, but failed to arrive. However, she attended the Diabetic Foot Clinic one month after that, walking in without an appointment. The amputation site was fully healed but nails had been pulled off all the lesser toes (Figure 1.25b).

Over the next 20 years she had numerous hospital admissions for infected neuropathic ulcers. Pulling pieces of skin off the heels eventually resulted in bilateral deep heel ulcers: these would heal in total contact casts but quickly relapse once the casts were removed, and it was clear that she was pulling pieces of tissue from the bases of the ulcers and the surrounding skin. She was seen by the Foot Clinic psychiatrist, but was unable to break the habit of pulling skin off her feet and remains with chronic neuropathic ulcers of both feet. She is aware that she is damaging her feet, but is unclear as to the motives behind this, and feels unable to stop. She has survived long term despite many ulcers and infections, and has no diabetic nephropathy and no cardiac problems.

Learning points

- Self-inflicted injuries can be a portal of entry for infection.
- Concurrent psychological problems make foot ulcers very difficult to treat.
- Self-inflicted ulcers are unrewarding to treat but care should never be withdrawn.
- Every diabetic foot clinic should have links with a psychiatrist as a member of the multidisciplinary team.

1.6 Long term patients followed in the Diabetic Foot Clinic with neuropathic foot problems

For many patients with neuropathic feet, long term attendance at a Diabetic Foot Clinic is the only way to avoid amputation.

Case 1.26   Long term management of a grateful patient who avoided losing his legs

---

The patient, a successful 40 year old banker, with Type 1 diabetes for 22 years, was referred to the Diabetic Foot Clinic after his local hospital proposed bilateral below knee amputations as the only solution to his indolent neuropathic ulcers. His feet had been ulcerated for over five years, and all his toes had been amputated during episodes of neuropathic ulceration complicated by infection. He had deep plantar ulcers on both forefeet five centimetres in diameter. However, X-ray did not reveal extensive osteomyelitis. The reason the local hospital gave for amputation was that they felt the ulcers would never heal and that unhealing ulcer is an indication for major amputation. This is a policy our Diabetic Foot Clinic has never adhered to. When told at his initial visit that his feet could be saved he wept with relief.

Initially he was treated with sharp debridement of his plantar neuropathic ulcers by the podiatrist (Figure 1.26a, b), and total contact casting. The ulcers became smaller and shallower, but after two months he developed infection of the left foot within the cast. There were no signs or symptoms until the cast was removed at a routine clinic appointment. There was oedema and crepitus in the soft tissues around the ankle, and X-ray revealed gas in the tissues. He was admitted the same day, and given IV amoxicillin 500 mg tds, flucloxacillin 500 mg qds, metronidazole 500 mg tds and ceftazidime 1 g tds. A tissue specimen taken in the Diabetic Foot Clinic grew anaerobic *Streptococcus*. His infection resolved over the next four days. In view of the problem under the cast, it was decided to discontinue total contact casting, and he was treated with regular podiatry to sharp debride the ulcers, felt padding to redistribute pressure from the ulcers, and orthopaedic boots with cradled insoles. He took prolonged courses of antibiotics. The ulcer healed (Figure 1.26c).

However, we were unable to achieve long term healing of the ulcers. The patient attended the Diabetic Foot Clinic for 17 years and his feet survived despite frequent episodes of ulceration and recurrent infections necessitating hospital admissions on nine occasions. By arrangement, most of these admissions were to his local hospital and were for acute sepsis, and on each occasion his CRP was very high, ranging between 188.3 and 371.6 mg/l. He never needed surgery and always responded quickly to treatment with IV antibiotics. On one occasion he had an ulcer on the lateral border of his left foot. He went to the bathroom in the middle of the night and knocked his foot on the bathroom door. The ulcer bled, and he and his wife were unable to staunch the flow. She took him to the local hospital casualty department, where it was found that he had fractured a small calcified

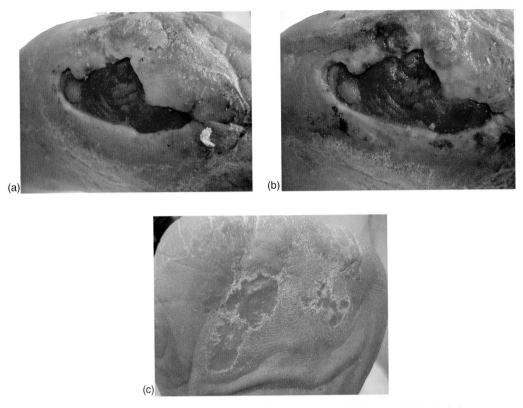

Figure 1.26 (a) Ulcer before debridement. (b) Ulcer after debridement. (c) Healed ulcer.

blood vessel within the wound bed. The leg was elevated and a compression bandage applied and the bleeding stopped. He was later referred to the dermatologists when he developed a cauliflower-like appearance of the skin on the dorsum of his foot. This was biopsied but no malignancy was found, and the dermatologists felt it was associated with long term lymphoedema of the foot.

Both his feet survived, despite recurrent episodes of ulceration and recurrent infections, for many years. He told us that he had weighed in the balance the benefits of having no ulcers against the benefits of leading an active life and doing the things he wanted to do, and he was convinced that whatever the future held he was not prepared to behave like an invalid and restrict his activities. We respected this decision. He eventually died of a stroke at home, having been unhealed for long periods, but always immensely grateful for the regular care that he received from the Diabetic Foot Clinic and the salvage of his feet.

Learning points

- Diabetic patients with neuropathy benefit from long term specialist follow-up care to treat their ulcers.

- It is impossible always to prevent recurrence of ulceration in many patients. The diabetic foot clinic needs to be available to receive and treat them.

- Patients with recurrent ulcers will get recurrent infections, which often need hospital treatment. However, neuropathic patients can often maintain mobility and remain free of major amputation. This patient had a long and successful career until the end of his life.

- A rare cause of haemorrhage in the neuropathic lower limb is a fractured calcified vein. This problem may lead to considerable bleeding. The leg should be elevated and pressure applied.

Case 1.27 Pain in the groin was this patient's warning sign of foot infection

Another lady with indolent neuropathic ulcers, whom we have followed over many years, was determined to live an active life and be independent.

This 40 year old lady with Type 2 diabetes for 5 years was referred to the Diabetic Foot Clinic 23 years ago with a deep infected ulcer – her first foot problem – and was admitted. She was a very house-proud housewife and always immaculately dressed. She had profound neuropathy, with a VPT of more than 50 V, and severe proliferative retinopathy requiring repeated laser therapy. At her first admission she needed a ray amputation for a deep plantar ulcer over the right fourth metatarsophalangeal joint with soft tissue infection and osteomyelitis. She stayed in hospital for three weeks and then attended the Foot Clinic regularly. She developed recurrent ulceration. After the right foot healed, she developed plantar ulceration on the left foot and needed amputation of the left first toe. During a subsequent episode of infection she lost her left fourth toe and had recurrent ulceration over several metatarsal heads. She then underwent resection of the remaining metatarsal heads on the left foot, which healed.

In total she had 20 infective episodes and needed six hospital admissions. She always insisted on removing her dressings at clinic visits herself, and putting them in the refuse bin without them being handled by staff. She also refused to use medical dressings on her feet, preferring to use round eye-makeup-removal pads, and brought a supply to clinic visits for dressing her feet. Her sight was not good enough for her to check her feet, and she was reluctant to ask her husband to do this, saying that she did not want him to see the ulcers in case it upset him. She never allowed him to accompany her to the Clinic but always drove herself there. The warning sign she relied on as a signal that she should come to the Foot Clinic in emergency was pain in the groin from lymphangitis. Despite her difficulties in checking her feet and detecting problems early, she has so far avoided major amputation, although she has frequent plantar ulcers (Figure 1.27) but leads an active life.

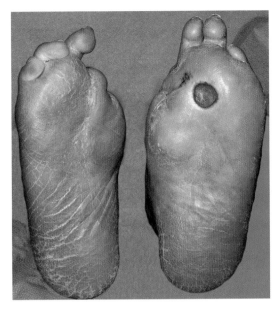

Figure 1.27   Healed minor amputations on both feet and plantar ulceration on the left foot.

Learning points

- Patients with neuropathy are vulnerable and need long term care.

- People with peripheral neuropathy are always susceptible to trauma and then infection, but can usually avoid major amputation if they seek specialist help in time.

- Partially sighted patients with proliferative retinopathy may not be able to see their feet and detect cellulitis early.

- Some patients have unusual ideas about wound care and dressings, which should be accommodated by staff wherever possible, as patients like to feel in control.

Case 1.28   "One damn thing after another"

A 37 year old man with Type 1 diabetes of 23 years' duration had a long history of plantar callus and neuropathic foot ulceration and was among the first patients treated at the King's Diabetic Foot Clinic. Initially he was issued with bespoke shoes with cradled insoles; his ulcers were regularly debrided and he did well until children at the school where he worked as a caretaker mocked him for wearing bespoke shoes and he decided to stop wearing them any more. Over the next three years he lost three lesser toes to septic vasculitis and infection, and this overloaded his plantar forefoot even more. He was very reluctant to take time off work and his in-patient admissions occurred during the school holidays, as during term time, except for routine monthly appointments outside school hours, he did not attend the Clinic. He developed a large deep ulcer with a diameter of more than three centimetres over his right first metatarsal head. This was only healed after a surgical procedure closed it through a racket incision (Figure 1.28a, b), but he then developed an ulcer over the fourth metatarsal head and said that he seemed to get "one damn thing after another".

The ulcer was healed after a period in a total contact cast during the long Summer vacation, but the foot broke down again within three months. The second toe had retracted and drifted laterally, and after a particularly busy time at work loading furniture his third metatarsal head area broke down (Figure 1.28c). He then agreed to wear a pair of bespoke shoes, so long as these were made to look "as normal as possible", and he was given a pair of blue and white trainer-style shoes with toe filler and cradled insole. His ulcers improved but he refused treatment with a total contact cast, saying that the foot would "just break down again" as soon as he came out of the cast. The head teacher at the school became very worried about him and suggested that he might consider taking early retirement. He became anxious about this, and accepted treatment with a living human skin equivalent, Dermagraft, and the ulcers healed within three months (Figure 1.28d).

He was encouraged by this and agreed to attend more frequently so that the callus on his feet did not have time to build up, and agreed with the Foot Clinic staff on a two week interval between treatments. Around this time, his wife began to accompany him to the Clinic. She asked questions about the pathogenesis of foot ulcers and the association between neglected callus and tissue breakdown, and she encouraged him to continue to attend the Foot Clinic more frequently. He had three years without ulceration. He then developed Charcot's osteoarthropathy in his left foot, and would not agree to treatment with a total contact cast until the foot had already developed a rocker bottom deformity. This was because it had been decided at the school that it would be dangerous for him to undertake his work while wearing a cast and he was still reluctant to take sick leave in case it was decided that he was unfit to work. Eventually a large plantar ulcer developed over the rocker bottom deformity (Figure 1.28e) and his wife persuaded him that the time had come to give up work, and he accepted early retirement on health grounds at the age of 54. The ulcer healed in a total contact cast; he continued to attend the clinic very regularly and to seek help at the first sign of any problem, and he did very well for the next seven years, with only brief episodes of skin breakdown, which were reported early and healed quickly. During this time he and his wife enjoyed several holidays abroad. She continued to work.

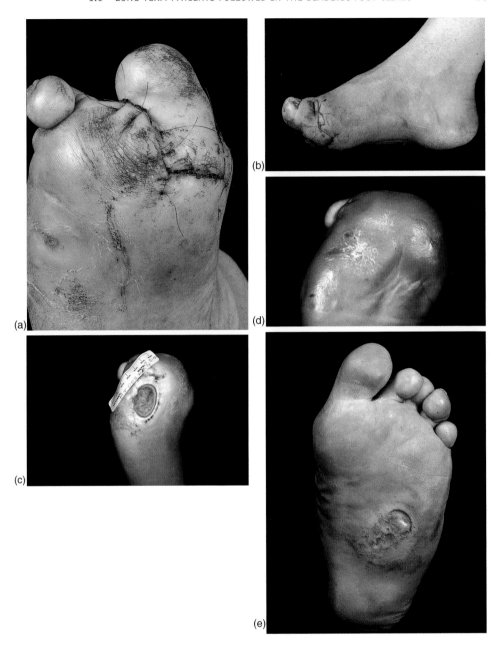

Figure 1.28   (a) Postoperative view of the right foot. (b) Lateral view. (c) Breakdown over the third metatarsal head. (d) Ulcer healed after application of Dermagraft. (e) Ulcer over rocker bottom deformity left foot.

When he was 61 years old, he developed unilateral oedema in his left leg, an abdominal mass was detected, he underwent laparotomy in another hospital and died on the operating table from uncontrollable bleeding.

Learning points

- This case study demonstrates again that, without effective offloading, plantar ulceration is very difficult to prevent and heal.

- Patients may be very sensitive about the appearance of their hospital footwear and every effort should be made to achieve a "normal" look.

- There are many different techniques that can be used to prevent and treat neuropathic ulceration, but the most important may be a change in the patient's lifestyle that enables him to rest the feet. Support from other family members is very useful and they should be encouraged to attend the foot clinic with the patient and to become involved in the treatment.

Case 1.29   Late onset neuropathic ulceration

Another of our original Foot Clinic patients had Type 1 diabetes and was a patient of Dr RD Lawrence.

This patient first presented at the Diabetic Foot Clinic at the age of 60 years with a deep long standing plantar ulcer complicated by osteomyelitis (Stage 4 foot). His Type 1 diabetes was diagnosed during World War II and he was a patient of Dr RD Lawrence at King's. Throughout his diabetic life, the patient's wife used a Lawrence metal template to measure out his portions of bread. This man worked on a building site. He had proliferative retinopathy treated with laser. He was admitted and underwent surgical debridement of the right foot. After three weeks of bed rest, the foot healed. However, he was doomed to almost continuous recurrences of ulceration. His left foot was less involved.

He had several admissions for infected neuropathic ulcers (Stage 4 feet). On one occasion, after his infection was under control, he was treated with Dermagraft and healed. However, the foot broke down again after four months. It was noted at the age of 83 years that his pedal pulses were no longer palpable and as he had further tissue loss he underwent angiography. There was diffuse disease of the superficial femoral artery but no significant narrowing. The anterior tibial artery and peroneal arteries were patent with no significant stenoses. He did not undergo angioplasty and the ulcer improved while he was in hospital.

He was becoming increasingly frail and during the last year of his life he had six admissions to hospital. He was first admitted with a deep necrotic heel ulcer, which grew MRSA, which was treated with teicoplanin 400 mg daily IM. Two months later, he had a recurrence of the heel ulcer, which became sloughy and probed to bone. MRSA was grown from the foot and he went home on teicoplanin 400 mg IM daily. After a further three months, he had an admission for diarrhoea and vomiting, thought to be caused by his antibiotics. The foot grew MRSA and *Enterobacter* species. He was treated with amikacin 7.5 mg/Kg/bd and teicoplanin 400 mg IV daily. Two months later, he developed dysphagia and weight loss. A barium swallow showed multiple tertiary contraction in the entire oesophagus. He also had ultrasound of the kidney and bladder, which showed significant residual volume after micturition, with 351.6 mls pre micturition and 222.5 mls post micturition. His serum creatinine was normal at 89 μmol/l. The heel ulcer was growing *Enterobacter* species and *Klebsiella aerogenes* and he was treated with IV amikacin 7.5 mg/kg bd and meripenem 1 g tds.

His penultimate admission was precipitated by a chest infection. His creatinine had risen to 144 μmol/l, CRP was 67.7 mg/l and a chest X-ray showed that he had volume loss in the right lower lobe with peribronchial thickening, indicating right lower lobe infection possibly secondary to aspiration. He treated with IV meropenem 1 g bd. By the time of discharge, his creatinine had fallen to within normal limits at 108 μmol/l and CRP was 6.2 mg/l.

However, he was back in hospital within a month, for his last admission. He was brought in after a severe hypoglycaemic episode during which he had aspirated. He developed pneumonia. X-ray showed right basal shadowing indicative of infection. His CRP rose to 96.0 mg/l and creatinine to 213 μmol/l. His WBC was 11.16×10^9/l, with neutrophils of 9.16×10^9/l. He was treated with meropenem 1 g bd but died on the ward of right basal pneumonia, at the age of 84 years. He had lived with Type 1 diabetes for 55 years and members of the Diabetic Foot Clinic were invited to and attended his funeral.

Learning points

- Although this patient had had diabetes for most of his life he was afflicted by neuropathic ulcers for the last 24 years. The diagnosis of his original neuropathic ulcer with cellulitis was delayed and this led to considerable osteomyelitis. Although the infection was treated and resolved, the patient had recurrent episodes of ulceration and sepsis in that foot.

- Indolent neuropathic ulcers can respond to adjunctive treatment such as Dermagraft, which is an artificial dermis which is applied directly onto the ulcer.

- Despite modern diabetic foot care, neuropathic patients often suffer from recurrent foot ulceration. Such patients need ready access to a multi-disciplinary diabetic foot clinic throughout their life.

- We have noted a pattern of increasing fragility in diabetic neuropathic patients as they reach old age, with frequent admissions to hospital from the Diabetic Foot Clinic, heralding their eventual demise. The Diabetic Foot Team have an important role to support patients and carers through this difficult period. Cure may not be possible but relief of symptoms and making patients comfortable should be a priority.

Case 1.30   Long term follow-up needed, at home, at work and on holiday

Patients with neuropathic feet can never relax, and can never afford to forget about their feet. A long term patient, discovered this on holiday.

One of the first patients to be seen in the King's Diabetic Foot Clinic was a 50 year old Afro-Caribbean lady with Type 2 diabetes of 10 years' duration. At a routine annual appointment at the Diabetic Clinic, a research fellow investigating diabetic peripheral neuropathy asked her to remove her shoes so that he could measure her VPT. She had a neuropathic ulcer on the apex of her left hallux, of which she was unaware. The ulcer was surrounded by heavy callus and discharging pus (Stage 4 foot) (Figure 1.30a). The skin on both her feet was very dry with cracking and fissuring around the heels. The VPT was 35 V and the pedal pulses were full and bounding. Dorsal veins were distended. The ankle brachial pressure index was 1.82. The podiatrist debrided callus from around and over the ulcer, advised use of an emollient to the areas of dry skin around the heels and arranged to see the patient every two weeks for further debridement. Negative casts of both feet were taken and the patient subsequently provided with two pairs of shoes with cradled insoles. The patient returned two weeks later, having rested at home with feet elevated in the meantime, and the ulcer was much improved (Figure 1.30b). After a further two weeks the ulcer had healed (Figure 1.30c) and the patient was given her new shoes, and offered monthly appointments at the Diabetic Foot Clinic, which she accepted.

Four years later she went on holiday to the West Indies and walked barefoot on the beach. As soon as she returned to the UK she attended the Foot Clinic as an emergency with an infected left hallux and a healing neuropathic ulcer on the dorsum of the left fourth toe. In view of the associated warmth and oedema and unusually poor diabetic control she was admitted to hospital for bedrest and IV antibiotics. She was discharged after one week with complete resolution of warmth and swelling. The ulcers were fully healed in one month. She was followed for the rest of her life and had a further episode of ulceration aged 65 years when she dropped a dustpan onto her foot and developed an ulcer on the apex of her second toe, which healed in one week. This problem was detected early by the patient, who attended the Diabetic Foot Clinic as soon as she noticed it at her daily foot inspection. She worked as a domestic cleaner until the age of 65 years.

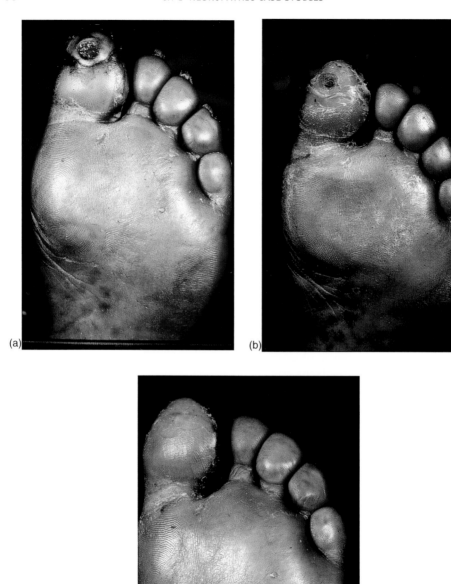

Figure 1.30 (a) Neuropathic ulcer on apex of toe. (b) Healing ulcer. (c) Healed ulcer.

Learning points

- Without inspection of the feet, neuropathic ulcers may not be detected because of lack of protective pain sensation, poor vision and unawareness of the feet.

- Neuropathic ulcers usually heal quickly with regular debridement of callus and rest and offloading and control of infection. Good shoes and insoles can help to prevent relapse.

- A change in environment often puts people with neuropathy or ischaemia at risk of foot problems.

- Patients who go on holiday are particularly vulnerable to trauma. One of the authors went on holiday with seven people, none of whom had diabetes and all of whom developed small foot problems, including blisters, deep fissures, traumatic injuries from wearing sandals, cuts from rocks in the sea and on the beach, and sea urchin spines in the feet. Because none of these people had neuropathy they were all aware of the problem, treated it, and healed without problems. Diabetic people on holiday often find it difficult to obtain specialist treatment locally even if they become aware of a problem.

- Long term outcomes can be very good in patients with a history of neuropathic ulceration so long as they have the services of a diabetic foot clinic and rapid access in emergency. When the neuropathy is profound then it is almost impossible to prevent occasional injuries to the feet, but, although ulcers cannot always be prevented, as in this case, they respond to treatment if caught early.

Case 1.31 Bathroom surgery

Self-treatment is best avoided if the feet are neuropathic. Bathroom surgery to remove callus led to ulceration in this lady.

A 54 year old lady with Type 2 diabetes for two years who worked as a domestic cleaner was referred to the Diabetic Foot Clinic by her general practitioner when she developed an ulcer on the sole of her foot (Stage 3 foot). The patient was aware that she had "a corn" and had been accustomed to shaving it with one of her husband's razors, but desisted when the foot "began to weep" and sought help. She had never received any foot care advice and had never attended the hospital Diabetic Clinic. She had a VPT of 40 V and bounding foot pulses. Her eyes had not been inspected for many years and she needed laser treatment for proliferative retinopathy. Her creatinine was 120 μmol/l and her glycated haemoglobin was 9%. She was referred to the Diabetic Clinic for her diabetic control to be improved.

Her right foot had a plaque of callus over the second metatarsal head with a small sinus connecting with an underlying ulcer (Figure 1.31a). The callus was removed to expose the true dimensions of the ulcer, and the patient was shown a digital photograph of the foot and was very disconcerted by the appearance of the ulcer. She was reassured that healing could be achieved, and was very cooperative with a proposed regime of bespoke shoes with cradled insoles, regular debridement of callus from around the ulcer and antibiotics to control infection. An X-ray showed no problem with the underlying metatarsal head. She was reluctant to give up work, but agreed to rest as much as possible. Her husband had taken early retirement from work and he was very supportive and agreed to undertake all of the domestic chores until her foot was better. She attended the Foot Clinic every week for debridement (Figure 1.31b). The foot healed in fourteen weeks (Figure 1.31c). She did not relapse and is alive and well 17 years later, still wearing bespoke shoes and attending the Foot Clinic regularly, and with good renal function and acceptable glycated haemoglobin levels.

The patient and her husband wanted to go to Majorca in the summer. When they first decided that they would like to do this they asked the Foot Clinic staff whether it would be wise and what special precautions they would need to take. (Since 1990 we have conducted a special "Holiday Footcare Programme" because of the high incidence of foot problems in people with diabetes who go on holiday. Many injuries are caused by the strange and unfamiliar holiday environment, extremes of climate, and burns and cuts from walking barefoot on beaches and in the sea. Moreover, some patients become so "light-hearted" when on holiday that their usual protective footcare regimes are relaxed and injuries are common.) She was warned to wear plastic sandals on the beach and in the sea, not to walk barefoot in the hotel room, to avoid sitting in hot sunshine, and not to discard her hospital shoes. She was advised to telephone the Diabetic Foot Clinic if any problems arose and to take a small first aid kit with her on holiday, containing antiseptic, dressings, bandages and tape. The holiday was very successful and the patient and her husband decided to return to Majorca the following winter for three months. She was then given the contact details of a podiatrist who practiced in Majorca, so that she could obtain regular preventive foot care, reduction of callosities and cutting of nails, and also

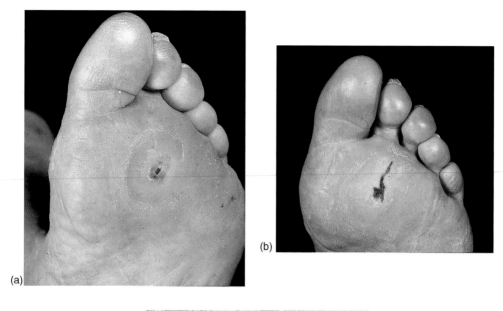

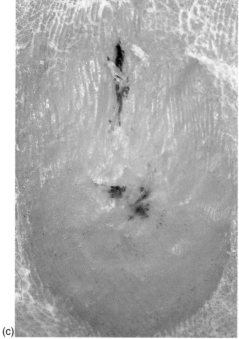

Figure 1.31   (a) Ulcer with callus. (b) The ulcer has been debrided. (c) Healed ulcer.

obtain local help if needed in emergency. The longer trip did not cause problems and now they always winter abroad.

Learning points

- In addition to looking at the feet, the Foot Clinic needs to ensure that good metabolic control is achieved.

- The support of the patient's husband helped her to continue working while achieving healing of the ulcer.

- Long term outcomes can be very good in patients who take their feet seriously and follow advice.

- Holidays can be hazardous for high risk diabetic patients. They should be carefully forewarned of possible dangers and told how to obtain help if problems arise.

- Many UK trained podiatrists work abroad and can see patients privately, if needed. The UK Society of Chiropodists and Podiatrists maintains a register of these practitioners.

Case 1.32   Contact dermatitis

A 76 year old widowed lady with Type 2 diabetes of 12 years' duration lived alone, but spent part of the year staying with her married daughter (who also had Type 2 diabetes) and son-in-law and their two children. She was very overweight with a body mass index of 32, and suffered from hypertension. Her diabetes was managed by the general practitioner and the practice nurse. She was determined to maintain her independence and never to become a burden to her family. She was a very cheerful and happy lady, who always chatted to staff and other patients about her grandchildren, and brought in home-made cakes as gifts. She believed that her diabetes was mild and "not really a problem. I just need to watch what I eat". Her diabetes was diet controlled.

She first came to the Diabetic Foot Clinic because while shopping one morning she knocked the front of her ankle on a supermarket trolley. She felt no pain at the time of the injury, but another shopper saw that the leg was bleeding and pointed it out to her, and a first aider at the shop cleaned the laceration and applied a dressing. When the patient returned home she applied further first aid. She filled a plastic bowl with warm water, mixed in half a bottle of Savlon antiseptic and soaked the foot and ankle for half an hour. The next morning the entire foot and lower leg were red and weeping. She applied gauze and a bandage and visited her general practitioner, who referred her to King's. Her VPT was 35 V and pedal pulses were palpable. The skin of her left foot and ankle was red, moist and weeping, with numerous small bullae (Stage 2 foot). She told us that she had tested the temperature of the water in the soaking bowl with her elbow and was sure that it was not hot enough to burn her foot. She was seen by the dermatologists, who felt that the problem was a contact dermatitis, due to an allergic reaction to the strong solution of Savlon (Figure 1.32).

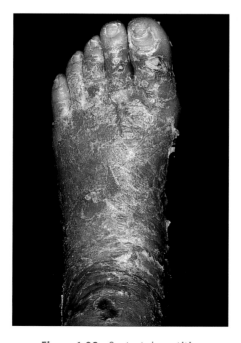

Figure 1.32   Contact dermatitis.

She was a advised to apply calamine lotion daily to the red areas. A district nurse called on her every day to check the foot and re-dress the laceration. Within a week the foot was dry and desquamating, and she made a good recovery.

In view of her neuropathy she was offered foot care and attended the Foot Clinic regularly. She then began to find the journey to and from the hospital difficult and did not want ambulance transport or a hospital car to take her, so treatment was sought from the community podiatry service and a podiatrist called at her home every three months. This was also arranged for when she was staying with her daughter.

Learning points

- All people with diabetes should be advised to seek professional help if they injure their feet.

- First aid for superficial injuries should be confined to cleaning, dressing and covering the wound with a dry dressing held in place by a loose bandage.

- The Diabetic Foot Clinic is not only a clinic but also a club, in which patients and staff form strong bonds of mutual comfort and support through good times and difficult times.

- Antiseptics should be carefully diluted in accordance with the instructions on the bottle.

Case 1.33 Colour change in the Afro-Caribbean foot

A 66 year old Afro-Caribbean woman with Type 2 diabetes of 22 years' duration was referred to the Diabetic Foot Clinic with swelling and discolouration of her left fourth toe (Stage 4 foot) (Figure 1.33). She had neuropathy with VPT of 29 V. Pedal pulses were palpable. She said that she had never received any help with her feet and cut her own toenails. She was awaiting operation for bilateral cataracts and her vision was poor. She was aware that she might have cut the flesh of the toe the previous week because she had seen a spot of blood on her white socks when she washed them, but could not see any problem with the foot until several days later, when she thought the toe was swollen and visited her general practitioner and was sent to the hospital. The medial sulcus of the toe was very swollen, with a splinter of nail penetrating the sulcus. Pus was drained and sent for culture, and she was given amoxicillin 500 mg tds and flucloxacillin 500 mg qds orally. *Staphylococcus aureus* was grown. The nail splinter was removed together with a small wedge removed from the side of the nail so that it would not press on the sulcus. The toe was cleansed with Hibitane in spirit and a dry dressing was applied. The district nurses were asked to visit her every day to check and redress the foot. At review after one week the toe was healed.

She was offered regular foot care, which she accepted, and attended the Foot Clinic for many years. Because her feet were not deformed and she had no callus or history of

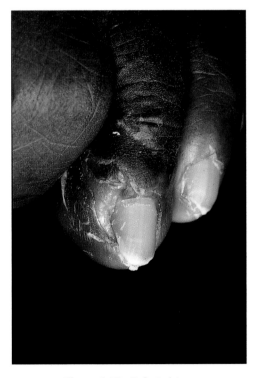

Figure 1.33 Infected toe.

ulceration it was felt that bespoke shoes were not needed. However, she received careful footwear education and was advised to wear lace up shoes with low heels for everyday and for around the house, and agreed to do this. She lived with her husband and an unmarried daughter, both of whom also had diabetes and attended the Foot Clinic and were very supportive. Despite stalwart attempts to control her diabetes as well as possible, her glycated haemoglobin levels gradually rose, and despite high doses of oral hypoglycaemic agents it was not possible to achieve optimal control and she was started on insulin.

She developed a plantar wart on her right heel at the age of 73 years and needed reassurance that treatment was not necessary so long as the lesion was painless and not spreading, and after two years it resolved spontaneously. Her skin was dry and she was encouraged to use an emollient and liked cocoa butter, which her daughter also used. She died at the age of 83 years of a stroke.

Learning points

- Colour change in the Afro-Caribbean foot with infection may be subtle but careful inspection will usually detect it.

- Patients with neuropathy should not be expected to cut their own nails.

- A frequent problem is caused when the patient cuts the flesh of the toe instead of the nail, or does not cut the nail completely, leaving behind a splinter of nail that penetrates the sulcus as the nail grows forward.

- Light coloured socks can often reveal a foot problem because blood or exudate forms a discoloured patch.

- Patients with new foot discolouration should be seen as an emergency on the same day the problem is first noted.

- High risk patients benefit from long term follow-up in a specialist centre.

Case 1.34   Sudden death

When patients with neuropathy appear young and healthy, active and cheerful, it is easy to forget how serious their problems are. The following patient appeared fit and well, remained in full-time employment, and then died very suddenly, without warning and without prior complaint of any problem.

A 46 year old man with Type 1 diabetes of 30 years' duration was a very early patient of the Diabetic Foot Clinic. He was referred to King's by his practice nurse, who reported that he had a blue right second toe and a neuropathic ulcer over the right second metatarsal head. He was not a local patient, coming from rural Kent, and all his previous care had been at the general practitioner's clinic, with annual visits to the diabetic department of his nearest district general hospital. He was profoundly neuropathic, with a VPT of over 50 V. His pedal pulses were full and bounding, the dorsal veins on both feet were distended and the plantar skin was dry and flaking. The neuropathic ulcer was deep to bone and the forefoot was cellulitic (Stage 4 foot). He denied ever previously receiving any foot care, or education relating to the feet, and had been unconcerned about "the hole in my foot" because "it did not hurt so it could not be anything serious, could it?". He had proliferative diabetic retinopathy, which had received laser therapy in his local hospital, and his vision was poor. When the redness and swelling of the forefoot was pointed out to him he said that he could not really see any difference between the two feet and had only been aware of the ulcer because his sock was always wet.

A diagnosis of spreading infection in the neuropathic foot was made and it was thought that septic vasculitis had led to occlusion of the digital vessels of the blue toe with septic thrombus. (At that time many practitioners believed that diabetic patients suffered from "small vessel disease", leading to the spontaneous development of black toes in feet with bounding pedal pulses, and it was often thought that nothing could be done for the patient apart from major amputation, which was an alarmingly common practice even in patients who were purely neuropathic with no macrovascular disease of the leg arteries.) He was admitted the same day and started on IV amoxicillin 500 mg tds, flucloxacillin 500 mg qds and metronidazole 500 mg tds and underwent a ray amputation. Tissue culture grew *Staphylococcus aureus* and Group B *Streptococcus*. The orthopaedic surgeon applied strips of sterile Vaseline-impregnated gauze around the foot to hold it together as much as possible but was careful not to prevent free drainage. It was his practice to cut through the strips so that if there was severe post-operative swelling they would not form a constricting band around the foot. Histology of the digital artery demonstrated that the arterial wall was invaded by white cells and the arterial lumen occluded by septic thrombus, thus confirming the suspicions of septic vasculitis as a cause of digital necrosis in the neuropathic diabetic foot. The foot was irrigated with Milton (2% sodium hypochlorite solution) four times a day, with great care being taken to wash the Milton solution off the surrounding skin and to apply emollient cream. A healthy glistening bed of granulation tissue formed within a week.

The patient was discharged, with crutches and a wheelchair, after three weeks, and followed as an outpatient in the Foot Clinic, but during his time on the ward he was carefully educated. When his wife visited him on the ward she was asked to come down to

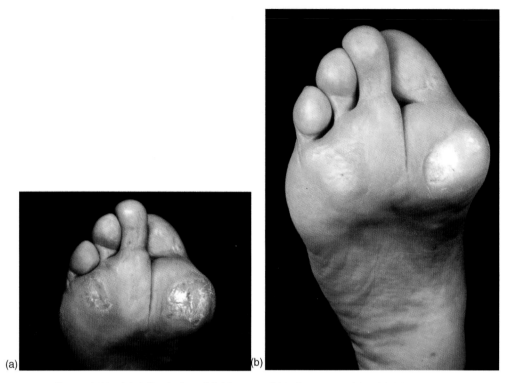

Figure 1.34 (a) Callus before debridement. (b) Callus removed by debridement.

the Foot Clinic with him, and we explained that due to his poor eyesight his feet were at risk and taught her how to perform a daily foot check, and she said that she would bring him to the clinic immediately if there was any change in the feet. She soon noted that he was developing heavy callus over the first and fourth metatarsal heads adjoining the ray amputation site (Stage 2 foot) and brought him to the Foot Clinic, where he underwent podiatric debridement of this callus (Figure 1.34a, b) to reduce the plantar pressures and prevent neuropathic ulceration. He was also reviewed by the orthotist at the next joint clinic and two pairs of bespoke shoes with cradled insoles were issued. His wife reported that he had found it very difficult to use the crutches to achieve complete off-loading because he frequently lost his balance and had to put his foot to the ground. She purchased a light-weight, folding wheel chair for him so that she was able to take him out and he did not become lonely, depressed and isolated. The foot healed quickly.

He had no further foot problems but died suddenly at work three years later. His wife came to visit the Diabetic Foot Clinic after his death and presented his wheel chair for the department's use

Learning points

- Infection of an ulceration over the metatarsal head can spread to the digital arteries of the adjoining toe, leading to septic vasculitis, occlusion of the arterial lumen by septic thrombus, and a black toe. If this is caught early and treated with antibiotics the process can be reversed: if the patient presents late, as in this case, loss of the toe is inevitable.

- After a ray has been removed, overloading of the adjoining metatarsal area is common. Regular removal of callus and offloading with an insole can reduce plantar pressures and prevent ulceration.

- Sudden death sometimes occurs in young neuropathic patients with no warning and is usually due to "silent" cardiac ischaemia.

Case 1.35   A cardiac arrest in the Diabetic Foot Clinic

Among our patients we have encountered sudden deaths both at home and in the hospital – and a "near miss" within the hallowed portals of the Diabetic Foot Clinic.

A 76 year old lady with Type 2 diabetes of 12 years' duration and known coronary vessel disease treated by coronary angioplasty at age 74 developed a sore on the end of her left second toe after she injured the flesh when cutting her nails. She visited her general practitioner when the toe became pink, and he arranged for her to see the practice nurse every week for dressings. She attended every week for four months, after which the toe became swollen and red. He then referred her to the Diabetic Foot Clinic. She had neuropathy, with VPT of 37 V. The pedal pulses were palpable. The toe was clearly infected with red fusiform swelling typical of osteomyelitis (Stage 4 foot): the so-called sausage toe (Figure 1.35). A small ulcer on the dorsum of the toe probed to bone, and an X-ray showed lucencies and erosions typical of osteomyelitis. She was reviewed by the orthopaedic surgeons but was very anxious that the toe should not be amputated if there was the slightest possibility of saving it and a trial of conservative care was agreed. A swab was taken from the ulcer, which grew *Staphylococcus aureus*. She was prescribed oral antibiotics with good bony penetration, namely fusidic acid 500 mg tds and doxycycline 100 mg daily, and these were continued for eight weeks, following which the ulcer had healed and the bony changes had improved on X-ray.

She was followed in the Diabetic Foot Clinic for the next two years. She was then admitted to hospital suffering from congestive cardiac failure. She improved and was sent down from the ward for a routine Foot Clinic appointment to have her nails cut and filed. After this procedure she was sitting in her wheelchair in the waiting room when the receptionist, who always keeps a close eye on patients, saw her head fall forward suddenly. The patient had lost consciousness and a podiatrist was called, who could not palpate her pulse. The patient was laid on the floor and cardio-pulmonary

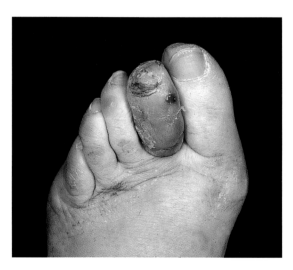

Figure 1.35   Sausage toe.

resuscitation (CPR) was commenced while the cardiac arrest team was bleeped. They arrived within two minutes and the patient was successfully resuscitated and moved to the Coronary Care Unit. She appeared to make a good recovery and was returned to the ward: however, two weeks later she had another cardiac arrest on the ward and could not be resuscitated.

Learning points

- Patients with breaks in the skin should be referred quickly for specialist care. Osteomyelitis can usually be prevented if infections are caught early and treated aggressively. This patient was kept under community care for too long.

- Osteomyelitis is the likely diagnosis in patients with "sausage toe", an ulcer which probes to bone, or when obvious bony changes are evident on X-ray.

- Osteomyelitis may respond to conservative care and amputation is not always necessary. Amputation of the toe is not always required in patients presenting with sausage toe. Management decisions are based on the clinical appearance, X-rays and the patient's wishes. Sometimes the response to antibiotics is very good and the ulcer heals, with complete resolution of the bone infection.

- When treating osteomyelitis conservatively, antibiotics with good bony penetration should be chosen.

- Diabetic foot patients are very frail. Many have multi-system disease. Our reception staff are instructed to keep a very close eye on patients in the waiting area. They get to know the patients well over the years, and are frequently the first to notice when a patient's behaviour is abnormal because of hypoglycaemia or when a patient is unusually pale or quiet.

- Patients should be closely observed at all times when they are at the Foot Clinic.

- All Diabetic Foot Clinics should have staff who are trained in cardio-pulmonary resuscitation (CPR) and a cardiac arrest trolley should be readily available. There should be a formal clinic policy relating to clinical emergencies so that when these arise all members of staff know what their roles are, i.e. who should call the cardiac arrest team and who should commence CPR.

Case 1.36   From neuropathic foot to ischaemic foot

We have included the last patient because he first presented as a pure neuropathic patient and subsequently developed peripheral vascular disease. The diabetic foot is a moving target.

This was a 30 year old patient with Type 1 diabetes for 16 years. He had bilateral proliferative retinopathy, bilateral cataracts and a previous retinal detachment, and his sight deteriorated so that he could not get a driving license. He was treated with bilateral photocoagulation. He attended the Diabetic Foot Clinic for many years with episodes of neuropathic ulceration and then attended in emergency, complaining that he had developed a small ulcer on the lateral border of his right fifth toe where he had never previously had an ulcer (Stage 3 foot). The ulcer had no surrounding callus and was in a "typically ischaemic" site, on the margin of the foot. His pedal pulses had become weak on the left and were impalpable on the right. He was admitted and underwent angiography. On the right there was a short segment occlusion at the level of the mid superficial femoral artery and a further short segment stenosis at the level of the right adductor canal; this narrowing and occlusion was angioplastied with a 5 mm balloon, and his ulcer healed in four weeks and did not recur.

Eighteen months later he complained of pain in his left calf when walking. He had angiography, which revealed disease of the left superficial femoral artery and a tight stenosis at the origin of the profunda artery. He underwent successful angioplasty and his claudication was relieved. Two years later he had a focal mid left superficial femoral artery stenosis of 70% and had another angioplasty. He continued to have episodes of ischaemic ulceration associated with infection for many years, but the ulcers quickly resolved. He died suddenly at home of a stroke ten years after his peripheral vascular disease was first diagnosed.

Learning points

- Diabetic patients with neuropathic feet can do very well, but only if they look after their feet well, seek help early, and receive multidisciplinary care when necessary.

- Neuropathic patients who are followed up may eventually become ischaemic. This process proceeds silently and may not manifest itself until the patient has developed ischaemic ulceration or gangrene.

- The burden of the neuropathic foot is great, both for patients and for health care professionals, but it becomes even greater when the neuropathic foot is complicated by ischaemia.

- Practitioners must be ever alert to the development of other diabetic complications apart from neuropathy.

2

Ischaemic Case Studies

2.1 Introduction

As we saw in the final case in the neuropathic patients chapter, during the course of patients' diabetic life, if they live sufficiently long, they are likely to develop ischaemia of the legs and feet. Nearly every diabetic patient with ischaemic feet will also thus have neuropathy, which is why we always describe these patients as "neuroischaemic". The combination of neuropathy and ischaemia is disastrous, and when treating diabetic patients with neuroischaemic foot we have been startled by the speed and subtlety of the natural history, and the wide range of comorbidities found. These neuroischaemic patients are supremely vulnerable and this must never be forgotten by those responsible for their care. Furthermore, by the time that the peripheral arteries are involved, the ischaemic patient is likely to have neurological and vascular impairment elsewhere.

If the Diabetic Foot Clinic takes on the management of diabetic ischaemic frail patients who will inevitably develop complications, the essential thing is to detect problems early and treat them optimally. If this can be achieved, most patients will do well in the end. There is no place for nihilism or ageism in their management. It is easy to find excuses for failure to act, such as the possibility that fragile patients will not survive vascular intervention, or the natural feeling that the elderly should be allowed to die in peace or that the patient has "had enough". However, we have been surprised by the positive long term outcomes when great efforts are made to salvage the neuroischaemic foot.

It is also important to be aware that neuroischaemic feet need long term care and scrupulously careful follow-up. Managing them is not a case of sorting out one acute problem and sending the patient away to live happily ever after. For the neuroischaemic patient, care by the Diabetic Foot Clinic must be a life-long commitment. It involves regular follow-up, routine preventive foot care, regular updating of education in order to avoid trauma and catch problems early, rapid and aggressive care of ulcers and necrosis, regular arterial and graft surveillance and the provision of statins and aspirin for secondary prevention of arterial disease. Thus, the long term follow-up care of the diabetic patient with peripheral vascular disease is an essential component of successful management, and staff, patients and administrators need to be aware of this. Patients with long term ischaemia need care that is readily accessible, specialised and enduring, which constitutes a long innings in a long game. Only excellent health care systems can deal successfully with

Diabetic Foot Care: Case Studies in Clinical Management   Alethea Foster and Michael Edmonds
© 2011 John Wiley & Sons, Ltd.

the diabetic neuroischaemic foot. The ideal forum for management of the acute episodes of infection and ischaemia is a combined vascular/diabetic foot clinic.

Patients with diabetic ischaemic feet are often under-estimated and under-treated, which is why the morbidity and mortality associated with diabetic foot is so high. The recent multicentre Eurodiale study highlighted the supreme vulnerability of patients with peripheral vascular disease: of all the diabetic foot patients treated in Eurodiale it was the patients with ischaemia and infection who had the worst prognosis.

The presentation of the neuroischaemic foot is unique: it differs from the classical picture presented by the ischaemic patient without diabetes and without neuropathy. Here, there is a natural progression through claudication, rest pain, ulceration and gangrene. Early signs and symptoms make the problem clear in the non-diabetic patient. However, the signs and symptoms of ischaemia in diabetic patients with concurrent neuropathy are much more subtle. Claudication and rest pain are not characteristic features and are often absent, and patients may initially present with tissue loss from either ulceration or gangrene. Furthermore, they do not have an intact autonomic system to regulate their homeostatic reflexes. Diabetic patients with ulceration who have the ominous combination of neuropathy and ischaemia are, therefore, supremely fragile. It is the presence of neuropathy together with ischaemia that confuses the picture not only in the foot but also in the rest of the diabetic foot patient, where even myocardial infarctions can be symptomless.

We were interested, when selecting case studies for this chapter, to see how many of the patients described have cardiac problems. Some of these heart problems were already known to be present – so many of our neuroischaemic foot patients have already undergone coronary artery bypass grafting that finding good veins to harvest for a leg bypass can be a problem – but other cardiac problems came to light only when they caused difficulties in patients undergoing vascular procedures to salvage the feet or in patients with infected ischaemic feet, where a bout of infection may have triggered cardiac failure.

In managing neuroischaemic patients, the Diabetic Foot Clinic at King's has passed from an era of conservative care in the earliest days of the Diabetic Foot Clinic in 1981 to modern and exciting developments of vascular techniques such as angioplasty, stenting, distal bypasses and the very successful hybrid procedures combining angioplasty and bypass. Bypasses last longer now with the modern trend to keep the bypass as short as possible, with much use of the various combinations of angioplasty and bypass (the so called "hybrid" procedures). There is increasing use of angioplasty also in conjunction with increased surveillance of bypasses, and when there is narrowing of proximal or distal ends of the graft it is dilated up with angioplasty. It is a rare occurrence now to find a patient who cannot be helped by angioplasty. Classically ischaemia in people with diabetes is distal below the knee, but it is not unusual for distal disease to be accompanied by femoral disease. Concomitant iliac disease is rare unless the patient is a smoker. It is important to treat the proximal disease first, as this will improve the flow in the distal regions.

Imaging techniques, such as non-invasive Duplex, have also changed the face of neuroischaemic care. We would like to deliver an additional very clear message: our experience is that very elderly and frail patients, including patients in renal failure, can benefit from vascular procedures, and even extreme old age is not a contra-indication to angioplasty or even distal bypass. Such techniques such as angioplasty and bypass should be employed to keep patients going, to preserve their legs and to improve their quality of life.

However, even today, with these technical advances now available, the importance of basic care (including early detection and control of infection) cannot be overestimated. For this reason, towards the end of this chapter we include some historic cases from the King's Diabetic Foot Clinic archive, of patients who were treated in the days before modern techniques were available, but who were helped by conservative care. We hope the lessons from these early cases will be helpful to practitioners in areas where high-technology procedures and investigations are not yet available. Our management of these patients, if seen today, would be much more aggressive, active and interventional than it was in the 1980s.

Notwithstanding major advances, the life expectancy of diabetic patients with peripheral vascular disease is still limited. It is best of all to keep patients ulcer free, but failing this early lesions should be treated aggressively. Sub-optimal treatment of small lesions in the neuroischaemic foot can lead to extensive tissue destruction needing major surgery, including debridement and bypass, and necessitating lengthy and debilitating stays in hospital. Thus, there is a need to see these lesions as early as possible and maintain them infection free if possible. However, infection remains "the great destroyer" of the diabetic foot, and to achieve success in dealing with fragile neuroischaemic patients the rapid management of any episodes of infection needs to be got right the first time with the assistance of modern microbiology. As several of our cases demonstrate, diagnosing infection can be difficult, especially when the signs and symptoms of infection are diminished by the presence of an all-pervading neuropathy.

Furthermore, treating infection in these patients is not just a matter of prescribing copious antibiotics: ischaemic feet need all the help they can get. Practitioners dealing with infection in the neuroischaemic foot should always seek out every opportunity for revascularisation, usually angioplasty, because improving the blood supply to the foot will also improve the foot's response to infection.

It is important to remember that patients who first present as neuropaths with bounding pulses will, if they live long enough, almost always develop peripheral vascular disease, and that if we succeed in preventing deformity and healing ulcers then the long term outcome will be better. Patients with acute Charcot foot are almost always neuropaths with good blood flow to the feet, but in years to come if they become neuroischaemic patients with chronic Charcot foot, and those feet have severe deformity, then management and prevention of ulceration will become very difficult.

As part of the approach to diabetic ischaemic feet, we should also not neglect the wound-healing opportunities provided by vacuum assisted closure (VAC). In the old days, agonising dilemmas would arise when an infection that clearly needed to be drained and debrided was present in a very ischaemic foot, which could not be revascularised and therefore had no hope of healing. Even when revascularisation is not possible, we have now found that by using VAC we can achieve healing of surgical wounds in extremely ischaemic feet.

We have also covered cases of people with widespread vascular disease who are nearing the end of their lives when no vascular intervention is possible. These people with end stage diabetes, end stage vascular disease and end stage feet need optimal care. Conservative care or palliative care does not mean leaving them to die as quickly as possible: it involves optimising their comfort, preserving a good quality of life and saving their legs if we can.

We found it a challenging exercise to divide up these neuroischaemic diabetic patients' case studies under specific subject headings, since their morbidities are so widespread and some of their histories are long and complex. The division headings we have chosen include

- Infection and its presentations

- Patients with severe co-morbidities

- Revascularisation
  Angioplasty
  Angioplasty and bypass
  Bypass

- Wound care

- Emboli

- Complications
  Angioplasty
  Bypass

- Pain in the neuroischaemic foot

- Conservative care.

Inevitably, in patients of such complexity, there are some areas of overlap, and some cases that could logically have been incorporated under more than one of the subject headings.

At this juncture, we wish to pay special tribute to the vascular surgeons and interventional radiologists at King's, and in particular to Hisham Rashid, Simon Fraser, Paul Baskerville, Huw Walters, Paul Sidhu, Jason Wilkins, David Evans and Dean Huang . We also feel deep gratitude to the Vascular Laboratory team of David Goss and Colin Deane and their colleagues, all of whom have worked tirelessly with our diabetic neuroischaemic patients for so many years, often at very short notice.

2.2 Infection and its presentations

As with all problems of the diabetic foot, catching things early is the key to successful management. This is the reason why, at King's, we do not believe in waiting lists for diabetic foot problems, and always aim to see patients within 24 hours if there is any break in the skin. It is easy to forget how very fragile some of our diabetic foot patients are.

Case 2.1   Systemic infection complicated by acute myocardial infarction and cardiac arrest

In the first case, there was an unfortunate delay before the patient sought help, and he was brought to Casualty by the emergency services. He was in very deep trouble within just a few hours despite intensive treatment of his infection.

A 66 year old patient, with Type 2 diabetes for 10 years, was an ex-smoker. He developed swelling, redness and pain involving the left first metatarsophalangeal area. This was originally a gouty tophus, which broke down and became infected (Figure 2.1a). There was a delay in presentation and the patient was ill on admission to Casualty with a Stage 4 foot. He also had significant co-morbidities with ischaemic heart disease and chronic obstructive airways disease. The CRP was 226.1 mg/l, uric acid was 0.56 mg/dl, and WBC was 13.71×10^9/l, of which 12.04×10^9/l were neutrophils. Serum creatinine was 103 µmol/l. MRSA was isolated from the foot cultures, and blood cultures also grew MRSA. Foot X-ray was normal. He was initially treated with IV vancomycin 1 g statim and then dosage as per serum levels, ceftazidime 1 g tds and metronidazole 500 mg tds, because he was allergic to penicillin in that he had previously developed a skin rash. Fourteen hours after admission to the ward he had a myocardial infarction and a ventricular fibrillation arrest, which was successfully cardioverted with DC shocks. He was resuscitated and intubated and ventilated on the Intensive Care Unit, and serum troponin was very raised at 27.21 µg/l (normal <0.05 µg/l). He had an echocardiogram, which showed multiple regional wall motion abnormalities. Left ventricular systolic function was severely diminished. He had two further episodes of ventricular fibrillation. He underwent coronary angioplasty, with insertion of two stents in the left anterior descending artery. He was put on antiplatelet therapy, consisting of aspirin and clopidogrel.

The foot lesion, infected gouty tophus, was debrided at the bedside and he continued on his IV vancomycin treatment. His peripheral vascular system was investigated. Doppler waveforms were damped and monophasic at the ankle, indicating that he had distal tibial disease. In view of his cardiac arrest and myocardial infarction it was decided to treat him conservatively and his foot lesion progressed satisfactorily (Figure 2.1b) and he is having long term follow-up in the Diabetic Foot Clinic.

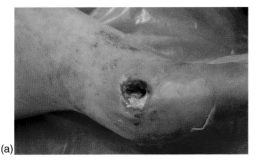 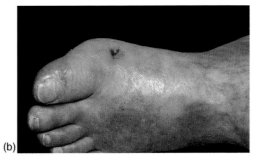

(a)   (b)

Figure 2.1   (a) Gouty tophus. (b) Healing foot lesion.

Learning points

- Patients admitted with ulceration may have serious comorbidities, which can be life threatening. This ischaemic man was ill and septic when he came in, and had a cardiac arrest soon after.

- Foot ulceration with sepsis is a medical emergency, especially in the ischaemic foot, and should be treated rapidly and aggressively.

- Gouty tophus can be a source of sepsis. Any break in the skin can be complicated by sepsis.

- This patient presented from the community with an MRSA infection.

- Community MRSA does not usually have the multiresistance of hospital acquired MRSA, but nevertheless can rapidly progress to severe infections. Approximately two-thirds possess the Panton–Valentine leukocidin (PVL) toxin, which acts to form pores in the cell membrane of mononuclear cells and polymorphonuclear cells and can lead to severe tissue necrosis.

- The acute infection in the diabetic foot and subsequent MRSA bacteraemia may have predisposed the patient to ventricular fibrillation.

Case 2.2   Severe infections: neuroischaemic patients are very susceptible to infection even after successful distal bypass

A 70 year old man, who had Type 2 diabetes for 9 years, hypertension, and gout, was seen in the Diabetic Foot Clinic with an infected sulcus to the right first toe. This was drained and debrided and he was given oral amoxicillin 500 mg tds and flucloxacillin 500 mg qds. This was a Stage 4 foot. A month later, he was admitted to hospital, when he presented to Casualty with shortness of breath and chest tightness, and in fast atrial fibrillation. He had a coronary angiogram that showed the left anterior descending artery to have 30–40% stenosis proximally. Distally, there was more diffuse disease with a right coronary artery 60–70% stenosis and a right circumflex artery 60–70% stenosis. He had angioplasty and multiple coronary drug eluting stents. He was considered for DC cardioversion but he had reverted spontaneously back to sinus rhythm.

Three months later he was admitted for infection of an ulcer over the right first metatarsophalangeal joint (Stage 4 foot) and *Staphylococcus aureus* was grown from the ulcer swab. This patient then underwent right femoral to posterior tibial artery bypass. Follow-up Duplex angiogram showed stenosis at the anastomosis of the proximal graft with the right femoral artery and clinically the patient had right foot pain (Figure 2.2a). He underwent

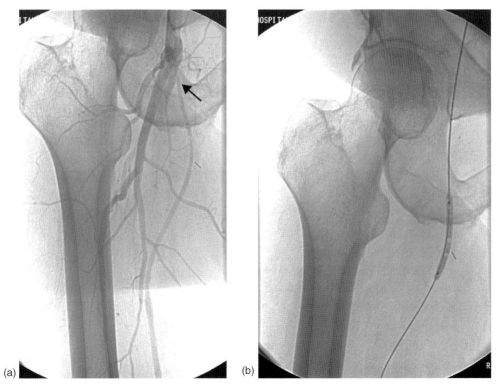

(a)   (b)

Figure 2.2   (a) Angiogram shows stenosis at the anastomosis of the proximal graft with the right femoral artery (arrow). (b) Balloon dilatation of the origin of the graft.

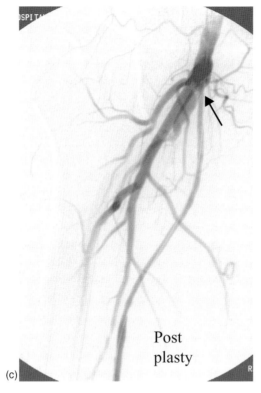

Figure 2.2 *(continued)* (c) Post angioplasty, showing resolution of the stenosis (arrow).

angioplasty of the origin of graft (Figure 2.2b, c) and his necrotic and infected right first toe (Stage 5 foot) was amputated. He had VAC therapy. The wound was healing well and a skin graft to the debrided toe amputation site was performed.

Follow-up surveillance with Duplex angiography showed monophasic pulsatile flow at the posterior tibial artery at the ankle and stenosis of the arterial graft in the mid-thigh with a threefold velocity increase. There was stenosis of the distal anastomosis with a five times velocity increase. An antegrade femoral angiogram was carried out, confirming narrowing at the distal anastomosis and tibial artery distal to the anastomosis. Further narrowing was also noted at mid-thigh level within the graft. The distal anastomosis and the distal vessel were dilated with a 3 mm balloon. The mid-thigh level narrowing was dilated with a 6 mm balloon. There was a good angiographic result.

One month later, the patient was readmitted with generalised weakness and fever. Group G *Streptococcus* was found in all four bottles of blood cultures taken on admission. A wound swab from the foot, where the wound was now very small, grew *Staphylococcus aureus* and Group G *Streptococcus*. He had a spiking temperature up to 40 °C. The patient was treated with IV co-amoxiclav 1.2 g tds which was later changed IV benzyl penicillin 2.4 g qds and flucloxacillin 1 g qds He had an echocardiogram to rule out endocarditis. A possible focus was the foot lesion; alternatively, given the relatively high grade bacteraemia, with organisms grown from every bottle, a cardiac source was thought possible. However, he had an echocardiogram, which showed no vegetations, so it was thought that the small wound on the foot was the source.

Learning points

- Every diabetic patient with a fever should have blood cultures.

- Patients with foot ulceration, however small, are prone to bacteraemia as the foot ulcer is a portal of entry and a foot ulcer need not be markedly infected to become a portal of entry of infection.

- This patient was regarded as having a high grade infection, as all four blood culture bottles grew Group G *Streptococcus.* No other source of group G *Streptococcus* was found apart from the foot ulcer.

- Patients having had distal bypass need intensive clinical follow-up preferably in a combined Vascular/Diabetic Foot clinic and also arterial graft surveillance in the Vascular Laboratory.

2.3   Patients with severe co-morbidities

Diabetic patients with multiple co-morbidities are a very complex group. Ischaemic foot ulcers may be precipitated and also aggravated by the presence of co-morbidities. Furthermore, vascular intervention may be complicated by the presence of co-morbidities, which may even prevent revascularisation from being carried out.

Case 2.3   Complex bypass in a patient with cardiac co-morbidity

This 78 year old man with Type 2 diabetes of 12 years' duration treated with insulin had ischaemic heart disease, and an implantable cardiac defibrillator for ventricular tachycardia. He was also on long term amiodarone and under close follow-up in the cardiac department. He was admitted with an infected left heel and ulceration of the first, second and third toes, and had critical ischaemia of the left leg. He had a cold left foot with ischaemic toes and necrosis of the second toe (Stage 5 foot) (Figure 2.3a). The feet were very swollen. Duplex angiogram of the left lower limb showed an occluded superficial femoral artery and proximal monophasic damped flow. Angiography revealed narrowing of the common femoral artery. There was blockage at the origin of the superficial femoral artery. The popliteal artery showed monophasic severely damped flow and the dorsalis pedis artery and posterior tibial artery were patent at the ankles with low flow and monophasic severely damped waveforms.

He was started on IV quadruple antibiotics amoxicillin 500 mg tds, flucloxacillin 500 mg qds, metronidazole 500 mg tds and ceftazidime 1 g tds. In order to optimise his cardiac condition, he had coronary angioplasty to the left main stem, left circumflex and the right coronary artery. He then underwent left and right renal artery stenting. This patient had an elective femoral to below knee tibio-peroneal bypass also with femoral endarterectomy (Figure 2.3b, c). The foot made good progress, with resolution of necrosis of the second toe (Figure 2.3d).

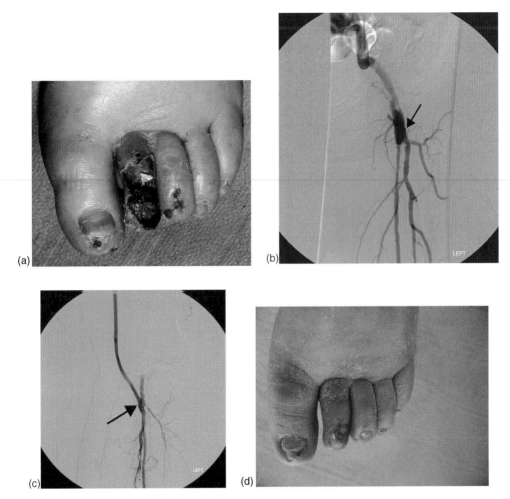

Figure 2.3 (a) Necrosis of second toe. (b) Proximal anastomosis of the graft (arrow). (c) Distal anastomosis of graft (arrow). (d) Resolution of necrosis of second toe.

Learning points

- Patients with cardiac co-morbidities need close management between the diabetic foot team and the cardiologists.

- Where possible, the cardiac function should be optimised, as in this case, with coronary artery stenting, before the patient undergoes peripheral vascular surgery.

- Having assessed and treated complex cardiac disease, there is no reason why it should rule out the possibility of distal arterial bypass.

- It is ideal to follow up these patients in a joint Vascular/Diabetic Foot Clinic.

Case 2.4   Neuroischaemic foot, gout and infection

This patient presented with gouty tophi on both feet, which precipitated ulceration in ischaemic feet.

A 78 year old man with Type 2 diabetes, impaired renal function with creatinine of 178 µmol/l, and gout, developed foot ulceration from gouty tophi over the medial aspect of both first metatarsophalangeal joints (Figure 2.4a, b). The ulcer on the left foot became infected(Stage 4 foot). His CRP was 37.1 mg/l. He was given IV amoxicillin 500 mg tds, flucloxacillin 500 mg qds, metronidazole 400 mg tds and ceftazidime1 g bd, later narrowed to flucloxacillin as *Staphylococcus aureus* was isolated. He was a smoker. He had a Duplex scan which showed a right superficial femoral artery occlusion and also an occlusion of the popliteal artery and stenoses in the posterior tibial artery.

He was not considered suitable for a day case angiogram in view of his impaired renal function, so he was admitted, and given N-acetyl cysteine 600 mg bd 24 hours before and 24 hours after his angiogram. On the right side the profunda artery was patent but with some disease proximally. There was proximal superficial femoral artery disease with diffuse disease running to the mid-thigh, where there was an occlusion of 8.6 cm reforming to a patent above knee popliteal artery. However, the popliteal artery occluded below the knee with reconstitution of the proximal posterior tibial artery via collaterals. The posterior tibial artery ran below the ankle and supplied a reasonable arch. On the left side there was a diseased profunda, and diffuse superficial femoral artery disease with occlusion of almost 10 cm in the adductor segment (Figure 2.4c). There was a good popliteal artery from above the knee with a tibioperoneal trunk but an occluded anterior tibial artery. The posterior tibial artery and peroneal artery were of poor calibre proximally but distally the posterior tibial artery ran across the ankle and formed an arch to the foot.

There was an attempt at subintimal angioplasty of the left superficial femoral artery but owing to the heavy calcification this could not be achieved and he was scheduled for a left sided distal bypass. However the infection responded to antibiotics and the ulcer on the left foot improved. He then developed infection of the ulceration on the right foot. He went to theatre and was on the operating table for a scheduled right distal bypass but not yet under general anaesthetic when he complained of chest pain and became short of breath. The procedure was cancelled. His blood troponin I was raised at 0.42 µg/l, indicative of myocardial infarction.

The patient developed fluid overload with impaired left ventricular function. His ECG showed partial right bundle branch block with lateral T wave inversion. He was given IV frusemide and his shortness of breath improved. He had an echocardiogram, which showed severely impaired left ventricular function with ejection fraction of 33%. His anterior, posterior and inferior walls were hypokinetic and his apex was akinetic. He underwent coronary angiography. The left anterior descending artery was diffusely diseased with moderate to severe proximal stenosis. The intermediate coronary artery had moderate mid-vessel disease. The circumflex artery was diffusely diseased, with a tight proximal stenosis and a further tight distal stenosis. The right coronary artery was small and subtotally occluded proximally with tight stenosis in the mid-vessel and distally. The

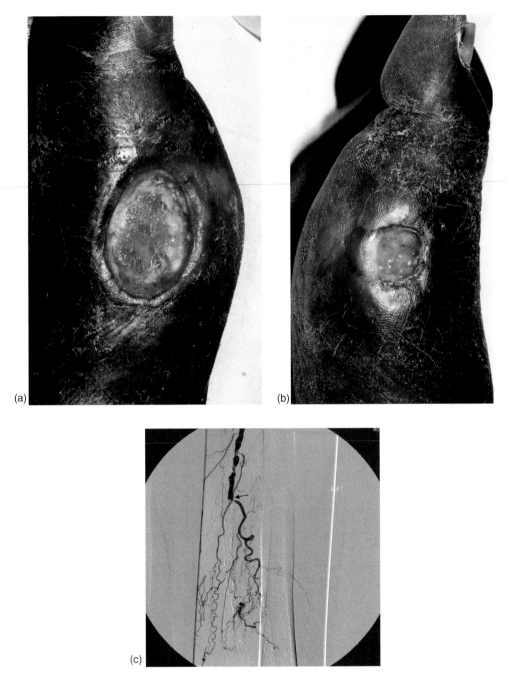

Figure 2.4   (a) Ulcer medial aspect of left first metatarsophalangeal joint. (b) Ulcer medial aspect of right first metatarsophalangeal joint. (c) Occlusion of left superficial femoral artery (arrow).

infection in his left foot eventually responded to antibiotics and in view of this response it was decided not to proceed with an arterial bypass as originally planned. It was decided to treat his coronary arterial disease medically. The ulcers were also treated conservatively and were slowly healing.

Learning points

- Once these patients develop infection in an ischaemic foot, they need very close supervision to continually assess the need for revascularisation.

- It is often said that diabetic patients characteristically have tibial artery disease, but profunda and superficial femoral artery disease are often present.

- When admitted to the hospital, diabetic ischaemic patients need close supervision as inpatients, regarding their cardiovascular state.

- This patient had virtually silent cardiac disease until he presented with a myocardial infarction just before his planned arterial bypass.

Case 2.5   Complicated neuroischaemic patient with autonomic dysfunction

This patient's co-morbidities also included heart problems, but in addition his bladder was affected by neuropathy, leading to urinary retention and greatly increased risk of urinary tract infection.

This was a 53 year old Type 1 diabetic patient with bilateral treated proliferative diabetic retinopathy, bilateral macular fibrosis and poor eyesight, who presented with left heel ulceration (Stage 4 foot) (Figure 2.5a). He had an eGFR which was 73 ml/min. He also had autonomic neuropathy as indicated by his postural hypotension and diabetic diarrhoea. He had undergone a right femoropopliteal bypass nine years previously, following an episode of severe sepsis in the right foot. He had also undergone popliteal angioplasty of the left leg. On this admission, he had left femoral angiography (Figure 2.5b). A focal distal popliteal stenosis was dilated with a 4 mm balloon with a good result (Figure 2.5c). The anterior tibial artery was a single vessel which supplied the ankle and foot (Figure 2.5d).

Whilst on the ward, he had episodes of hypotension and syncope. He had no chest pain but did have a serum troponin rise, indicating that these were episodes of acute coronary syndrome. Subsequently, coronary angiography showed moderate left main stem disease with severe proximal left anterior descending arterial disease and a subtotally occluded right coronary artery. He was felt to be a high risk candidate for conventional coronary artery bypass graft or angioplasty and it was decided to treat him medically. The patient continued to have hypotensive episodes associated with a rise in serum troponin. Synacthen test showed his steroid reserve to be normal.

One month after discharge, he had a further admission for infection of the left heel ulcer (Stage 4 foot). He also had a further episode of hypotension but no chest pain, and serum troponin was again raised. His heel cultures grew ESBL *E. coli* and he was treated with IV meropenem 1 g bd, and he improved and was discharged. Two months later, he was admitted in urinary retention and infection. He had presented to the Diabetic Foot Clinic again with a history of shivers and rigors. He had a raised CRP and blood count with neutrophilia. Urine showed nitrites and leucocytes. An ultrasound scan showed large post-micturition volumes. The bladder ultrasound showed normal kidneys but a distended bladder with residual volume of 431 ml post micturition. A neuropathic bladder was diagnosed. The patient was catheterised and given IV gentamicin 210 mg as a stat dose. The urine grew ESBL *E. coli*, which was sensitive to meropenem and gentamicin. He was treated with meropenem and then started on long term nitrofurantoin with regular urinary catheterisation. However, he had recurrent urinary tract infections, and was treated with IV meropenem at home through a PICC line.

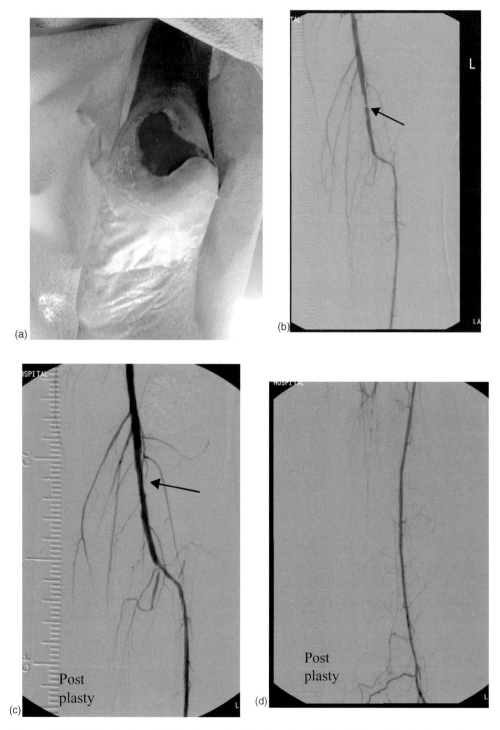

Figure 2.5 (a) Heel ulcer. (b) Angiography showing stenosis in left popliteal artery (arrow). (c) Dilatation of popliteal stenosis (arrow). (d) Anterior tibial artery supplying ankle and foot.

Learning points

- This patient had severe autonomic neuropathy and did not have chest pain when he had acute coronary syndrome.

- A diabetic patient with autonomic neuropathy and a prolonged period of hypotension should be suspected as having hypotension of a cardiac origin. Although patients with autonomic neuropathy can drop their blood pressure as part of their postural hypotension, a prolonged period of hypotension whilst supine may indicate an acute coronary syndrome and the patient should have a serum troponin measured.

- The patient had bladder urinary retention with an easily palpable bladder, but the patient complained of no discomfort. There was also no discomfort in his feet associated with ulceration. We have seen several cases of patients with painless ulceration and painless distended bladders from urinary retention and call this presentation the foot/bladder syndrome.

- This patient illustrates the vulnerability of the diabetic foot patient, with widespread arterial disease, widespread neuropathic disease and diminished eyesight.

Case 2.6   Ulceration in a neuroischaemic patient with cryoglobulinaemia

This man's ulcers were multi-factorial in their aetiology and not solely related to peripheral arterial disease. However, ischaemia needed to be addressed before healing could be achieved

A 55 year old man had Type 2 diabetes controlled with diet alone. He had a history of Raynaud's, with high rheumatoid factor and cryoglobulinaemia. He also had Sjögren's syndrome, hepatitis C, and peripheral neuropathy and peripheral vascular disease. He was treated with interferon alpha 2a and ribavirin. He developed ulcers on both feet, which were therefore at Stage 3. One ulcer was on the dorsum of the right foot, with a similar lesion on the dorsolateral aspect of the left foot (Figure 2.6a, b). His ulcers were punched out and circular. It was not clear whether the ulcers were due to peripheral vascular disease or his co-morbidities. He had initially an MRA, which showed that iliac, femoral and popliteal arteries were normal. On the right, below the knee, there was a short occlusion of the proximal peroneal artery. Distal to this, the peroneal artery was

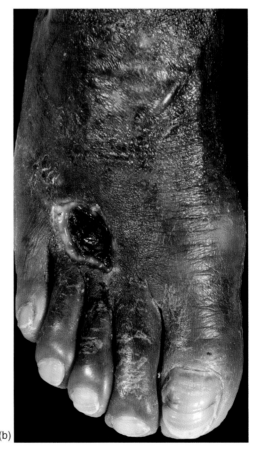

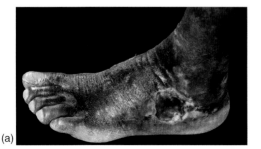

(a)   (b)

Figure 2.6   (a) Ulcer on dorsolateral aspect of left foot. (b) Ulcer on dorsum of right foot.

patent and the posterior tibial and anterior tibial arteries were diffusely and markedly diseased. On the left, there was a similar appearance of widespread tibial disease but the dorsalis pedis artery was patent bilaterally.

The ulcers deteriorated and he was treated with piperacillin/tazobactam 4.5 g tds IV. The ulcer swabs grew *Staphylococcus aureus* and group G *Streptococcus* and the therapy was changed to IV amoxicillin 500 mg tds and flucloxacillin 500 mg qds. He initially underwent a left popliteal to posterior tibial artery bypass. He then had a right femoral angiogram, which showed occlusion of the posterior tibial artery. The peroneal artery was occluded and reconstituted as a single vessel to the plantar arch via the posterior tibial artery. The anterior tibial artery was diseased at the proximal aspect and occluded a short distance away. A 2 mm balloon was used to dilate this area. The occlusion was not crossed. He therefore underwent distal bypass from popliteal to dorsalis pedis on the right. His ulcers gradually improved and healed.

Learning points

- This man's ulcers were multi-factorial in their aetiology and not solely related to peripheral arterial disease. The Raynaud's, cryoglobulinaemia and interferon alpha 2a probably contributed.

- However, the peripheral arterial disease contributed to the poor healing of these ulcers, and blood flow to the feet needed to be improved to aid healing. The only way to do this was by distal arterial bypass.

- We have seen increasing numbers of patients who have a pattern of distal arterial disease below the knee. Sometimes, these patients are not frankly diabetic: they have normal fasting glucose but impaired glucose tolerance. They must be managed as if they are diabetic patients and may need distal revascularisation, if feasible.

- This man's diabetes was treated solely by diet: another so-called "mild" diabetic patient in deep trouble.

Case 2.7   Necrosis in a patient with antiphospholipid syndrome

Severe widespread ischaemia is seen in the antiphospholipid syndrome (thrombophilia). This case describes a patient with this syndrome who developed necrosis.

This lady with Type 2 diabetes presented with a painful ischaemic, necrotic, right second toe (Stage 5 foot) (Figure 2.7a) as well as severe pain in the right thigh for four days, worsening over the previous 24 hours. In the past, the patient had had positive cardiolipin antibodies, and a diagnosis of antiphospholipid syndrome had been made. She had had a previous right femoral embolectomy and a middle cerebral artery infarct.

The patient was treated with warfarin and the INR should have been maintained between 3 and 4. However, prior to this presentation, the patient had developed haematuria and her INR had fallen. Duplex angiogram showed the superficial femoral artery and common femoral arteries to be occluded on the right (Figure 2.7b). Thus there was an exacerbation of the antiphospholipid syndrome, resulting in an acute thrombo-embolic occlusion due to INR being sub-therapeutic at 1.93. She was treated with enoxaparin sodium as an anticoagulant and also aspirin. Her foot swab grew *Enterobacter aerogenes* and she was treated with IV meropenem 1 g tds, to which it was sensitive. The right second toe became dry and the tip auto-amputated. Regarding her haematuria, she had a normal cystoscopy and CT urogram and the haematuria eventually resolved spontaneously.

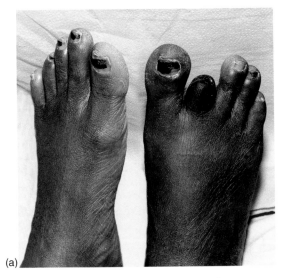

(a)

Figure 2.7   (a) Necrotic right second toe.

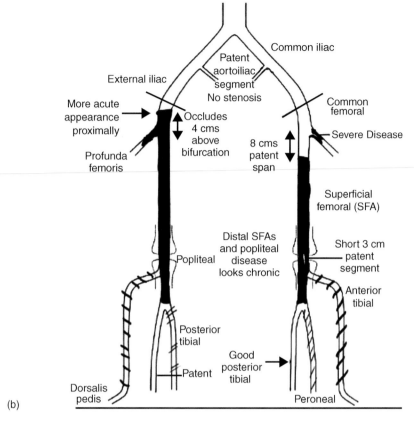

Figure 2.7 *(continued)* (b) Diagrammatic representation of Duplex angiogram, showing occlusion of superficial femoral artery and common femoral artery on right and superficial femoral artery on left.

Learning points

- Patients with diabetes may develop thrombotic conditions such as the antiphospholipid syndrome, which aggravate the large vessel arterial disease of diabetes and present with episodes of thrombosis throughout the arterial tree.

- It is important to measure phospholipid antibodies and to diagnose the antiphospholipid syndrome, as the results of surgery are poor in this syndrome and early anticoagulation is important.

- Diabetic patients with peripheral vascular disease and other conditions such as antiphospholipid syndrome need very careful follow-up in the multidisciplinary Diabetic Foot Clinic.

Case 2.8 HIT syndrome – heparin induced thrombocytopenia

Superadded vascular disease may sometimes be caused by therapy. We describe a distressing case of a lady with thrombocytopaenia induced by treatment with heparin.

A 63 year old lady with Type 2 diabetes presented as an emergency in the first few years of the Diabetic Foot Clinic with an ulcerated infected right third toe and blueish discolouration of the right foot (Stage 5 foot). She was obese and her diabetes was poorly controlled, with glycated haemoglobin of 10%. The foot was pulseless and Doppler studies revealed a pressure index of 0.42. She was admitted to hospital and treated with IV antibiotics and unfractionated heparin. An arterial bypass was not possible due to lack of run-off. The patient's necrosis spread and she underwent a major amputation of the right leg below the knee.

The patient developed a low platelet count and the amputated stump of the right leg and the remaining left foot became severely ischaemic. Heparin induced thrombocytopenia thrombosis syndrome (HITTS) was diagnosed. Heparin was stopped but the patient continued to have widespread thrombosis and died.

Learning points

- Heparin induced thrombocytopenia (HIT) can present in two forms. Type 1 is a mild non-immunological process associated with high dose IV heparin related to mild direct platelet activation by the heparin acoride chain. Type 2 HIT leads to a greater fall in platelet count, with a greater than 50% decrease.

- The likelihood of Type 2 HIT is substantially greater for unfractionated heparin rather than low molecular weight heparin. When it is severe, it leads to heparin induced thrombocytopenia thrombosis syndrome (HITTS). This involves active thrombus formation, which is severe and life threatening. Thrombosis occurs when platelet thrombi develop at sites of pre-existing pathology and lead to thrombus formation.

- A low platelet count and unexpected clinical events of thrombosis should raise the diagnostic possibility of HITTS.

- The treatment of HIT and HITTS is difficult. The use of additional heparin is contra-indicated in the presence of heparin mediated thrombosis.

- It is now possible to perform reliable anticoagulation in HITTS with preparations such as leprudin and avoid increasing the risk of thrombotic events.

2.4 Revascularisation

2.4.1 Angioplasty

The next seven cases illustrate the value of angioplasty, including repeated angioplasty, in treating a range of lesions caused by various injuries in ischaemic feet. These include injuries caused by footwear and bathroom surgery. Angioplasty of the arteries of the leg including the tibial arteries is established as the initial definitive procedure in revascularising the diabetic ischaemic foot, even in the most elderly of patients.

Case 2.9 Diabetes, liver transplant and angioplasty

A 64 year old man with Type 2 diabetes of 26 years' duration was referred to the Diabetic Foot Clinic with a necrotic left fifth toe (Stage 5 foot). He had chronic renal impairment from diabetic nephropathy and had undergone a liver transplant seven years previously. He had had a right below knee amputation at his local hospital. He was admitted to hospital and given IV antibiotics amoxicillin 500 mg tds, flucloxacillin 500 mg qds, metronidazole 500 mg tds and ceftazidime 1 g tds.

His CRP was only 6.7 mg/l but three days later the CRP had risen to 63.3 mg/l. A wound swab grew *Staphylococcus aureus* and antibiotics were narrowed down to flucloxacillin. The toe was amputated, and a skin graft was applied to the wound. He underwent angiography. There was occlusion of the posterior tibial artery at mid-calf level and multiple narrowings of the mid to distal anterior tibial artery, and these lesions were angioplastied. Possibly because of his immunosuppression, his foot was slow to heal.

We then followed him at regular intervals. One year later, he had a myocardial infarction and a coronary artery bypass graft, herpes zoster associated with left upper arm paralysis, and then came back to the Diabetic Foot Clinic with an infected, necrotic left second toe (Stage 5 foot) (Figure 2.9a). The infected toe had been present for three weeks during which he had been convalescing at a local Cottage Hospital after his coronary artery bypass graft. His CRP was 259.6 mg/l, and WBC 11.97×10^9/l, with neutrophils comprising 10.12×10^9/l. He underwent digital amputation. (Figure 2.9b). He was treated with IV antibiotics again as above. Tissue from the toe grew MRSA and the antibiotics were changed to IV vancomycin 1 g stat and then according to serum levels. He also underwent angioplasty. There was no significant superficial femoral artery or popliteal disease. Below the knee the peroneal artery was the main vessel to the ankle. The anterior tibial artery occluded a few centimetres distal to the origin, as did the posterior tibial artery (Figure 2.9c). There was a dorsalis pedis artery in the foot filling via the peroneal. The anterior tibial artery occlusion was crossed and dilated to 3 mm, resulting in straight line flow into the foot via the anterior tibial artery (Figure 2.9d). The amputation wound healed well.

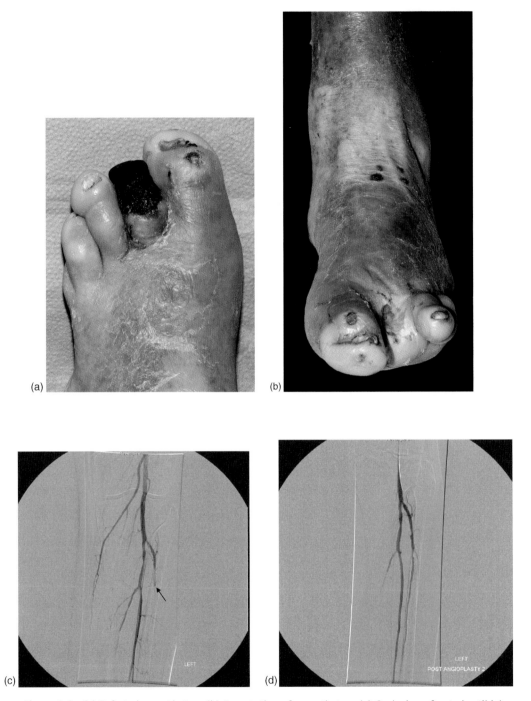

Figure 2.9   (a) Infected necrotic toe. (b) Amputation of necrotic toe. (c) Occlusion of anterior tibial artery (arrow). (d) Resolution of anterior tibial artery occlusion.

Learning points

- This patient's response to infection was impaired because of his liver transplant and immunosuppression and also his diabetes. Infections in his foot rapidly developed into digital necrosis.

- This needed aggressive management with IV antibiotic therapy, removal of the necrotic toe and urgent revascularisation.

- The serum CRP reflects inflammation from the previous 24 hours. On admission to hospital it invariably continues to rise for at least 24 hours and then should fall in response to therapy.

- Diabetic ischaemic patients who suffer intercedent illnesses such as myocardial infarction are at increased risk of recurrent foot ulceration and should have close preventative foot care on the coronary wards and during rehabilitation.

Case 2.10   Rapid deterioration

This 65 year old man had Type 2 diabetes for 10 years with peripheral vascular disease He had undergone a coronary artery bypass graft. He had rheumatoid arthritis treated with methotrexate. He was first seen at the Diabetic Foot Clinic when he was referred with a right necrotic hallux (Stage 5 foot) (Figure 2.10a). (Three weeks previously he had presented to Casualty with a painful right foot and angiography had demonstrated stenoses within the common iliac artery and superficial femoral artery, which were angioplastied, but the occlusion at mid-superficial femoral artery could not be crossed.) He was admitted and initially treated with IV antibiotics amoxicillin 500 mg tds, flucloxacillin 500 mg qds, metronidazole 500 mg tds and ceftazidime 1 g tds, which was then changed to oral amoxicillin and metronidazole in response to the isolation of Group B *Streptoccocus* and mixed anaerobes. He underwent a further right lower limb angioplasty of a focal superficial femoral artery stenosis with an eccentric plaque (Figure 2.10b). The stenosis did not respond to angioplasty so a 6 × 14 mm stent was placed with a good result (Figure 2.10c). The toe healed.

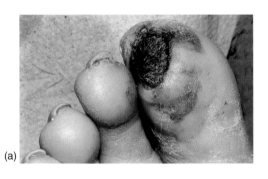
(a)

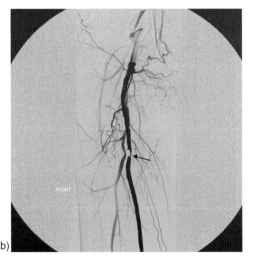
(b)

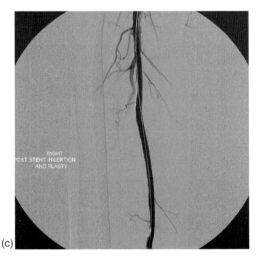
(c)

Figure 2.10   (a) Necrotic hallux. (b) Eccentric stenosis proximally in superficial femoral artery (arrow). (c) Superficial femoral artery with post-stent insertion.

Learning points

- It is important to note that this patient had deteriorated very quickly because of infection on the background of existing ischaemia.

- When he came to the Diabetic Foot Clinic he was admitted immediately and treated for infection whilst arrangements for urgent angioplasty were made.

- Stents are useful in the iliac and superficial femoral arteries, providing scaffolding of the vessel lumen, pushing plaque and vessel wall aside to enlarge the lumen when angioplasty fails.

Case 2.11   Angioplasty in a frail ischaemic patient

A 68 year old man with Type 2 diabetes of 31 years' duration had a cerebrovascular accident in India with a residual dense right hemiplegia and speech badly affected. He was referred to the Diabetic Foot Clinic the following year and offered regular foot care, as both feet were pulseless. Three years later, his family brought him to the Foot Clinic with an ulcer, which had a necrotic base on his right heel (Stage 5 foot). Both feet were pulseless. He was treated as an outpatient day case and underwent angioplasty of a focal area of stenosis in the right superficial femoral artery in the adductor canal. This was angioplastied with a 5 mm balloon. There was diffuse disease in the peroneal artery, which was also angioplastied with a 3 mm balloon and the heel ulcer improved.

Two years later, he developed necrosis and infection of the right fourth and fifth toes, with rest pain in the foot, and was admitted to hospital. Swabs grew *Morganella morganii* sensitive to meripenem and his antibiotic therapy was IV meripenem 1 g tds. During this admission he had an arterial Duplex, which showed a threefold velocity increase in the proximal common femoral artery and a further stenosis at the superficial femoral artery origin, with velocities greater than 3 metres/second. His CRP was 52.8 mg/l and white count 12.07×10^9/l, with neutrophils 9.54×10^9/l. He underwent right femoral angioplasty, and the necrotic toes were resected under general anaesthetic, after which he went into cardiac failure, developed bilateral pulmonary oedema soon afterwards, and went to the High Dependency Unit. He also developed pneumonia during this admission and his CRP peaked at 149.2 mg/l. His wounds were very slow to heal.

In a further admission for these wounds, which had deteriorated and become infected in the right foot, he underwent arterial Duplex on the right side but no common femoral artery stenosis was found. The superficial femoral artery and popliteal arteries were patent. However, foot specimens at that time were growing *Staphylococcus aureus* and *Morganella morganii* and he was given IV meropenem 1 g tds. The wounds healed.

Finally, he was admitted, very unwell, with a white count of 29.77×10^9/l with neutrophils 27.68×10^9/l and pneumonia, having come to the Diabetic Foot Clinic for a routine appointment. His chest X-ray showed perihilar airspace opacification with bilateral pleural effusions. He was treated with IV meropenem 1 g tds and recovered. His foot remains intact (Figure 2.11).

Learning points

- This patient is still alive after ten years of peripheral vascular disease. He is a very important member of his extensive family, who all adore him and come to the Foot Clinic with him whenever they can. His wife is always with him, and demands optimal care for him in every way. This is reflected in his long survival.

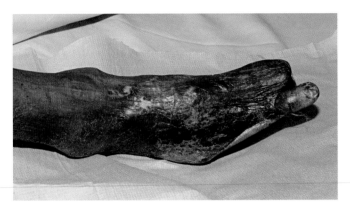

Figure 2.11 Intact foot.

- This patient illustrates the value of intensive long term care, keeping close surveillance of ulcers, postoperative wounds and the peripheral arterial tree in the Diabetic Foot Clinic.

- The patient had severe co-morbidities, with cardiac vessel disease and cerebrovascular disease, but the reverse is not the case, since many patients with coronary and cerebrovascular disease are free from peripheral vascular disease.

Case 2.12 Shoes with rough linings

A 60 year old man with Type 2 diabetes of 7 years' duration, diabetic nephropathy, diabetic retinopathy, autonomic neuropathy, peripheral sensory neuropathy with vibration perception threshold of more than 50 V and peripheral vascular disease with ankle brachial pressure index of 0.58 was referred to the Diabetic Foot Clinic from the Diabetic Department, where annual review had detected an ulcer on the apex of his right fourth toe. This was a Stage 3 foot. He believed the problem was caused by a rough place within his shoe where the lining was rucked up. The ulcer had the appearance of an ischaemic ulcer with a punched-out look and no associated callus (Figure 2.12a). He was issued with extra-depth shoes with cushioned insoles. A swab grew *Pseudomonas aeruginosa* and ciprofloxacin 500 mg bd was prescribed. He took early retirement from work on medical grounds.

The ulcer was very slow to heal and he developed another ulcer on the lateral border of the same foot. The toe ulcer was almost healed in 12 weeks (Figure 2.12b), but the marginated ulcer was still present after two years of conservative care. He then underwent angiography, which showed multiple stenoses of the popliteal and anterior tibial artery. The stenoses in the anterior tibial artery were dilated to 3 mm. Stenoses in the distal popliteal artery were dilated to 5 mm. After this intervention, the ankle brachial pressure index rose to 0.82 and the ulcer healed.

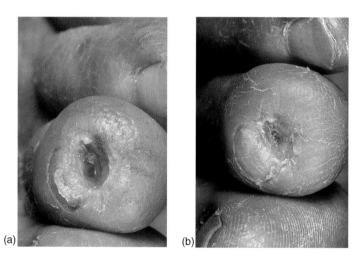

Figure 2.12 (a) Ulcer with the appearance of an ischaemic ulcer with a punched-out look and no associated callus. (b) The toe ulcer almost healed after 12 weeks.

Learning points

- At annual review the shoes and socks should always be removed.

- Patients should be taught to run their hands around the inside of the shoes before putting them on, in order to detect rough places.

- Extra-depth, wide-fitting shoes can reduce pressure on the vulnerable margins of the foot.

- Angioplasty should be explored in all cases of delayed healing.

Case 2.13   Bathroom surgery in an ischaemic foot

An 83 year old man with Type 2 diabetes of 19 years' duration was referred to the Diabetic Foot Clinic by his general practitioner. He had complained of discolouration of the toenails the previous year, with friable white patches. When his GP told him that it was a fungal infection and that treatment would be protracted and unlikely to succeed, the patient attempted an experimental treatment involving "bathroom surgery" to remove one of the nails. The toe began to bleed so the patient desisted from further "treatment".

A week later the right second toe began to turn black (Figure 2.13) and the patient showed the problem to his GP, who sent him to the hospital. The ABPI was 0.44. Balloon angioplasty of a popliteal occlusion was performed. The toe was amputated and the foot healed in one month. The patient refrained from any further treatments and attended the Foot Clinic every month, when his nails were filed and the thickness reduced.

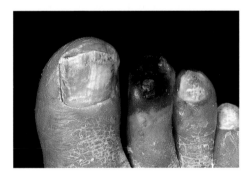

Figure 2.13   Necrotic tip of second toe.

Learning points

- Bathroom surgery is dangerous for patients with neuropathy or peripheral vascular disease and patients should be taught never to attempt self-treatment but to seek expert advice.

- If pulsatile flow can be achieved then gangrenous toes can be amputated, but in pulseless ischaemic feet a conservative approach, with eventual autoamputation of the black toe, may be applied. However, with the increasing use of VAC therapy toes may be amputated even in ischaemic feet that cannot be revascularised and healing of postoperative wounds still achieved with VAC therapy.

- Patients who have undergone a vascular procedure should be followed long term.

2.4.2 Angioplasty and bypass

The next group of patients underwent various combinations of angioplasty and bypass. Within this group, are patients who had specific hybrid procedures which combine angioplasty and bypass as integral parts of an overall strategy and are defined as follows:

Hybrid 1 – angioplasty before bypass,

Hybrid 2 – angioplasty after bypass,

Hybrid 3 – angioplasty with bypass.

Case 2.14 Purple toe

A 65 year old man with Type 2 diabetes of 14 years' duration was referred to the Diabetic Foot Clinic by his general practitioner complaining of a "purple" toe. There was no history of trauma. His vibration perception threshold was 23 V and his pedal pulses were palpable but very weak. He smoked 20 cigarettes a day. The distal two-thirds of the left first toe was deep purple in colour. The ankle brachial pressure index was 0.95. This was a Stage 5 foot. The lesion was thought to be embolic in nature and he was admitted to hospital and treatment with warfarin was commenced. He underwent angiography, revealing severe bilateral iliac disease, which was probably the source of his embolus.

There was severe disease within the left external iliac artery, with a near occlusive plaque. The left common femoral artery was patent and there was no specific common femoral artery or popliteal disease. At this stage there was a two vessel run-off with a patent anterior tibial and peroneal artery. A 7 mm × 6 mm and a 7 mm × 4 mm overlapping stent insertion was performed along the left external iliac artery. Angiography also revealed a right common iliac focal stenosis (Figure 2.14a) and angioplasty of the right common iliac artery was carried out with an 8 mm balloon (Figure 2.14b) (Figure 2.14c).

On discharge he was closely followed in the Diabetic Foot Clinic. The purple area developed dry necrosis and this was very gently and carefully debrided. Over the next five months the necrotic areas dried and were debrided away to reveal a healed toe with conservation of far more tissue than had been thought likely when he first presented, when he was warned that salvage of the toe was unlikely. He had received strong advice to give up smoking, and attended a smoking cessation clinic, but was unable to stop.

Six months later he had developed left foot ulceration and a downstream left sided angiogram revealed good inflow through the left iliac and femoral vessels, disease of the trifurcation and confirmed two vessel run-off. The ulceration did not heal and he underwent a left popliteal to posterior tibial bypass with eventual healing of the ulcer.

He then developed a necrotic right fifth toe and had a distal bypass and an amputation of the right fifth toe. Three months later, angiogram revealed occlusion of the right bypass graft. The right common femoral artery was balloon dilated to 6 mm and a re-do of his right bypass was carried out as a Hybrid 1 procedure. Postoperative angiography showed narrowing of the anastomosis distally and he had angioplasty as a Hybrid 2 procedure. He remains an irregular attender who smokes heavily.

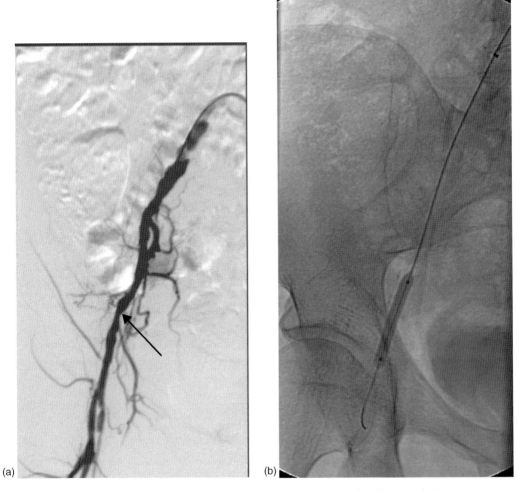

Figure 2.14   (a) Right common iliac focal stenosis (arrow). (b) Balloon angioplasty.

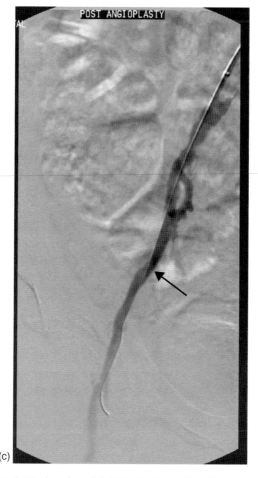

Figure 2.14 *(continued)* (c) Post balloon dilatation (arrow).

Learning points

- Embolism lodged in a digital artery leads to ischaemia of the toe with subsequent necrosis.

- The extent of the necrosis is difficult to determine in the early days and management should be conservative as salvage of much of the affected toe may be possible with good conservative care, as in this case.

- The patient underwent several combinations of angioplasties and bypasses as dictated by his clinical condition. This is the modern practical approach of combining these procedures rather than considering them as competing procedures.

- Nicotine is strongly addictive, and many patients are unable to stop smoking.

Case 2.15   Elderly man who underwent two successful distal bypasses

This man also underwent multiple procedures.

He was an 80 year old man who had Type 2 diabetes for 23 years. He was admitted with an ischaemic right foot and necrotic first toe. This was a Stage 5 foot. Angiography showed normal vessels down to the popliteal and on the right there was a patent peroneal supplying the foot. The anterior and posterior tibial arteries were occluded. There was a tight stenosis at the origin of the right peroneal, which was dilated to 3 mm (Figure 2.15a–c) but he did not have sufficient blood flow to allow amputation of the

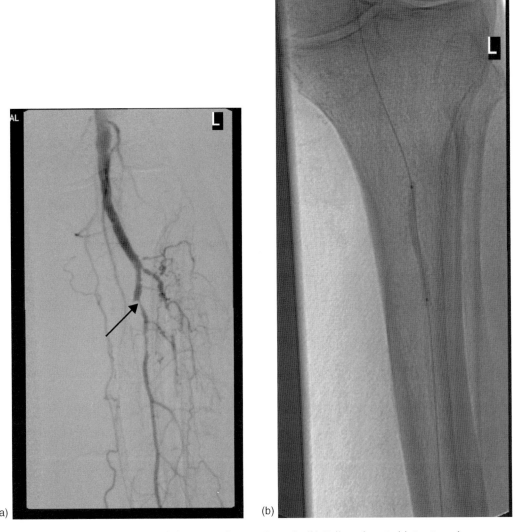

(a)   (b)

Figure 2.15   (a) Stenosis in peroneal artery (arrow). (b) Balloon inserted into stenosis.

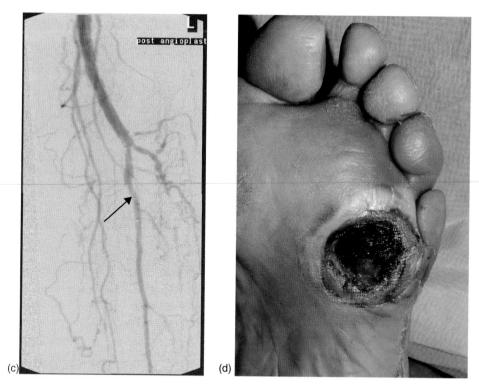

Figure 2.15 *(continued)* (c) Post angioplasty: the stenosis is dilated (arrow). (d) Ulcer on lateral border of foot.

hallux and be sure of healing of the postamputation wound. He underwent a popliteal to dorsalis pedis bypass on the right side and a right first toe amputation.

He then presented at the Diabetic Foot Clinic with an infected ulcer at the left fourth and fifth metatarsal heads with necrosis (Figure 2.15d). This was a Stage 5 foot. He was strongly advised that he needed immediate admission but he insisted on going home first to get his pyjamas, and failed to return. We were unable to contact him. The police were asked to check the house, and found him lying on the floor having fallen over and not being able to get up. He was brought to hospital, and admitted. His CRP was 129.6 mg/l. His creatinine was 207 μmol/l. A wound swab grew *Morganella morganii* and *Enterococcus faecalis* and he was treated with vancomycin and meropenem. He then had left sided popliteal to posterior tibial bypass. Initially the CRP rose from 107.6 to 155.8 mg/l but it subsequently fell to 118.6 mg/l. The rise was in response to his surgical operation. Graft surveillance revealed a thrombus at the distal end of the graft and he underwent successful angioplasty as a Hybrid 2 procedure and the foot healed well.

Learning points

- This elderly man underwent two successful distal bypasses. He developed peripheral vascular disease in his 80s and has been followed in this decade in the Diabetic Foot Clinic, needing angioplasties and subsequent bypasses.

- Although he had an angioplasty of his peroneal artery there was insufficient flow to heal the foot and thus he went on to distal bypass.

- He has had several episodes of infection associated with his ischaemia, which responded to aggressive antibiotic therapy.

- He now approaches his 90th birthday with intact feet.

Case 2.16 Osteomyelitis in a neuroischaemic foot

This case illustrates that elderly people can do very well.

A 90 year old lady with Type 2 diabetes for 25 years developed ulceration over the left first metatarsophalangeal joint, which was complicated by osteomyelitis, as shown by extensive destruction of the metatarsal head (Figure 2.16a). This was a Stage 4 foot. Her

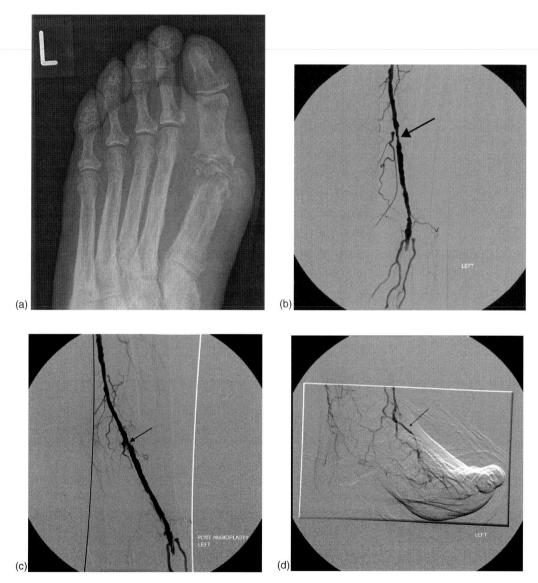

Figure 2.16 (a) Destruction of the first metatarsal head by osteomyelitis. (b) Narrowing in the superficial femoral artery before angioplasty (arrow). (c) Distal superficial femoral artery lesions have been dilated (arrow). (d) Angiogram showing run-off in foot and dorsalis pedis artery (arrow).

pedal pulses were not palpable. She underwent angiography, which showed diffuse disease of the superficial femoral artery with focal narrowings distally and occlusion of the popliteal artery. Initially she underwent angioplasty of the superficial femoral artery (as a Hybrid 1 procedure) but straight line flow to the foot was not achieved (Figure 2.16b, c). However, collaterals reformed a distal anterior tibial and dorsalis pedis artery. She was then considered for distal bypass. She was regarded as fit for this, having no cardiac symptoms and a normal ECG. She had a femoral to dorsalis pedis artery bypass (Figure 2.16d) and resection of the first ray and her foot healed successfully.

Learning points

- If the patient is fit, age is no bar to distal bypass.

- Initial angioplasty did not achieve straight line flow and thus distal arterial bypass was needed.

- It is difficult to manage osteomyelitis conservatively in a severely ischaemic foot.

- A ray amputation might not have healed without a successful bypass.

Case 2.17   Revascularisation and infection

This 80 year old man had Type 2 diabetes, and a CVA with a left fronto-parietal infarct and residual expressive dysphagia and known dementia. The patient was initially admitted with collapse. He had ischaemic heart disease and a previous myocardial infarction. The echocardiogram showed moderate valvular aortic stenosis.

He was admitted five months later after he developed infected ulceration of the right foot. This was a Stage 4 foot. Quadruple antibiotics were prescribed. He was given IV amoxicillin 500 mg tds, flucloxacillin 500 mg qds, metronidazole 400 mg tds and ceftazidime 1 g bd. The swab grew mixed anaerobes and his antibiotics were narrowed down to metronidazole. Doppler studies of the right leg showed significant tibial vessel disease and he underwent a right popliteal–posterior tibial bypass graft with amputation of the right fourth and fifth toes. The wound was post-operatively treated with VAC therapy and then underwent skin grafting. A Duplex angiogram the following month showed that the proximal graft was patent with slow flow. The posterior tibial artery distal to the graft demonstrated areas of focal narrowing (Figure 2.17a). The distal posterior tibial artery was dilated with a 2 mm balloon as a Hybrid 2 procedure (Figure 2.17b) with improvement (Figure 2.17c).

Two months later the patient was admitted again with right leg swelling. A deep vein thrombosis was suspected but ruled out. The foot had healed so infection was unlikely, and it was concluded that the oedema was normal post-bypass swelling. At graft surveillance two months later a Duplex showed that the graft was patent with good flows. He continued to have close surveillance. The foot remained healed.

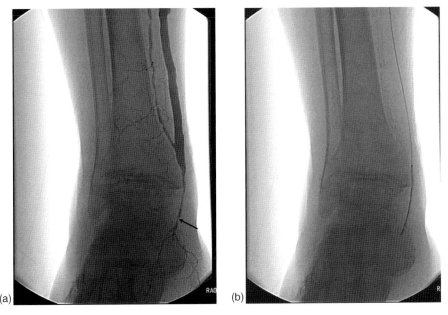

(a)   (b)

Figure 2.17   (a) Focal narrowing in posterior tibial artery (arrow). (b) Balloon dilatation.

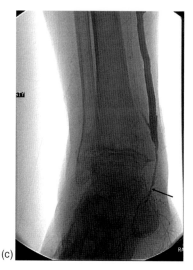

(c)

Figure 2.17 *(continued)* (c) Post angioplasty improvement (arrow).

Learning points

- Distal bypass grafts need extensive servicing and a close surveillance within a framework provided by the vascular laboratory.

- In the first year surveillance is performed at one week, then at one month, and then at each three monthly intervals thereon for one year.

- Oedema of the leg, after it has a bypass operation, is to be expected and is of venous and lymphatic origin.

- Cerebrovascular disease is not a contraindication to lower limb revascularisation.

Case 2.18 Angioplasty followed by bypass

A 78 year old man with Type 2 diabetes for 20 years underwent a below knee amputation of the left leg before he was referred to King's. He presented with ulcers over the medial aspect of the right leg and ankle and extending on to the dorsum of the foot. This was a Stage 4 foot (Figure 2.18a, b). Angiography demonstrated stenosis of the superficial femoral artery and the anterior tibial artery was occluded at the proximal third of the calf, but collaterals combined to form a single vessel at the distal third of the calf. He underwent angioplasty of his superficial femoral artery. Then he had a right popliteal artery to peroneal artery bypass (Hybrid 1 – angioplasty followed by bypass). He was closely followed up, with graft surveillance.

His ulcers were slow to heal. He had a further angioplasty later that year, and the following year he had a redo of the right sided peroneal bypass with a jump graft from his old graft to the distal artery. The ulcer persisted for six months, and he underwent a pinch skin graft to speed healing. The new jump graft had graft surveillance and a proximal stenosis was detected, and he underwent angioplasty and stenting with final healing of the ulcer.

He had recurrent infections in his ulcers. When first seen he grew *Pseudomonas aeruginosa*, which was treated with ciprofloxacin and gentamicin. Later, he grew *Stenotrophomonas maltophilia* sensitive to co-trimoxazole. He also grew MRSA sensitive to vancomycin, *E coli* sensitive to meripenem and *Alcaligenes* species sensitive to ciprofloxacin.

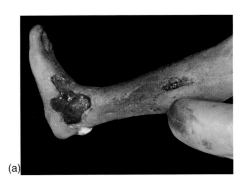 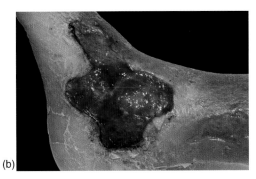

(a) (b)

Figure 2.18 (a) Panoramic view of leg. (b) Close-up view of foot.

Learning points

- This patient was nearly 80 years old when first referred to King's. He had already undergone a major amputation and the remaining leg was very precious, since although he was using a wheel chair he was able to transfer without assistance and thus retain some independence.

- Angioplasty of superficial femoral artery disease and distal bypass from popliteal to one of the tibial arteries or peroneal artery is a favoured Hybrid 1 approach to keep the length of the arterial bypass to a minimum.

- Long term follow-up, with early detection of problems, maintenance of optimal perfusion of the foot and rapid treatment of infected ulcers, was crucial to his successful management.

2.4.3 Bypass

The next group of patients all underwent arterial bypass. This is a major operation and patients need to be followed very closely, both in the peri-operative period and long term. We believe that results of bypass in diabetic patients compare very well with results in non-diabetic patients, but only if care is optimal and great pains are taken to act quickly if complications arise.

Case 2.19   Infected leg wound after bypass

An 81 year old lady with Type 2 diabetes for 10 years was admitted with necrosis of the right first toe. This was a Stage 5 foot. Angiography revealed no significant disease of the right external iliac or common femoral arteries. The superficial femoral artery occluded proximally a short distance from the origin. The superficial femoral artery reconstituted distally as a very poor vessel that then occluded. The profunda was of good calibre. The popliteal and trifurcation were occluded. There was a patent distal anterior tibial artery and dorsalis pedis. There were no suitable lesions for angioplasty.

The patient underwent a right femoral distal bypass. Vein was harvested from the left leg. The patient developed erythema of the wound of the left leg from which the vein had been harvested and purulent discharge occurred (Figure 2.19a). A deep swab showed growth of *Stenotrophomonas maltophilia* and *Escherichia coli*. The former organism was sensitive to co-trimoxazole and the E coli was sensitive to the trimethoprim. Both were sensitive to piperacillin/tazobactam, which was then given at 4.5 g tds IV. The leg wound healed (Figure 2.19b. Healed wound).

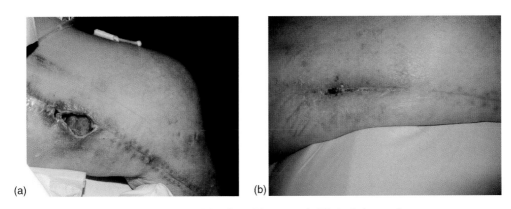

(a)   (b)

Figure 2.19   (a) Infected leg wound. (b) Healed wound.

Learning points

- Patients who have undergone a bypass need careful follow-up of their leg wounds.

- Swabs should be taken to ensure that antibiotic treatment is appropriate.

- *Stenotrophomonas maltophilia* can be a significant cause of soft tissue infection.

Case 2.20　Dressings should be lifted regularly to detect deterioration

This lady developed infection that was masked by a dressing.

A 62 year old Afro-Caribbean lady with Type 2 diabetes mellitus of 9 years' duration had peripheral neuropathy and proliferative retinopathy, which was treated with laser photocoagulation. Her feet did well for ten years after diagnosis in that she had never had a foot ulcer, and she checked her feet regularly for signs and symptoms of foot problems. At the age of 72 she attended as a self-referred emergency saying that she had visited the practice nurse with a small wound on the lateral aspect of her foot and a dressing had been applied. Her foot had "felt funny" for the past four days and was now "uncomfortable". Pedal pulses were impalpable and Doppler studies revealed an ankle brachial pressure index of 0.40. There was spreading infection from the lateral aspect of the foot through the plantar aspect (Figure 2.20a). This was a Stage 4 foot. The foot was debrided in theatre (Figure 2.20b). She underwent angiography and a distal bypass was performed the following day. After a skin graft was applied, the foot healed in three months (Figure 2.20c). This patient needed a three month admission to get her out of trouble. She survived, but the hospital stay was debilitating and her family said that she was never the same again.

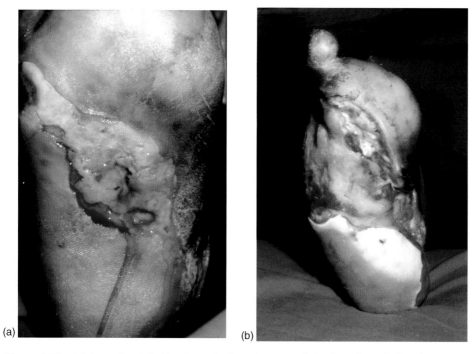

(a)　　　　　　　　　　　　　　　　　　　　(b)

Figure 2.20　(a) Spreading infection from the lateral aspect of the foot through the plantar aspect. (b) The foot post debridement.

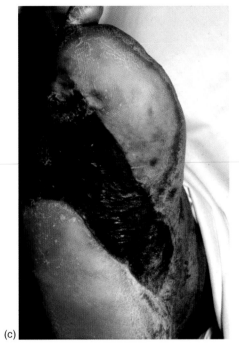

(c)

Figure 2.20 *(continued)* (c) Healing of foot after skin graft.

Learning points

- Ischaemia can develop silently in a previously neuropathic patient.

- Dressings can mask gangrene. Patients who lack protective pain sensation should have their feet checked every day.

- Dressings should be lifted to detect infection early.

- Patients with extensive tissue necrosis should undergo distal bypass to restore pulsatile flow and promote healing of these large deficits.

- Optimum treatment of ulcers in the neuroischaemic foot should avoid major infective complications and the associated lengthy hospital admissions.

Case 2.21   Episodes of acute ischaemia and infection

This man had a Stage 2 foot. Although there was no tissue defect, he was in deep trouble, with acute ischaemia of his left foot.

A 77 year old Afro-Caribbean man with Type 2 diabetes of 22 years' duration attended the Diabetic Foot Clinic after seeing the clinic sign in the hospital corridor. His left leg had become cold and very painful the previous day. The left leg had strong femoral pulses but none at the knee and the foot, and Doppler studies detected no blood flow in the foot. This was a Stage 2 foot with acute ischaemia. He was seen at once by the vascular surgeon, who performed an emergency distal bypass the same evening. The next day the foot was warm and swollen with palpable pedal pulses. The leg wound took four months to heal and he attended the Foot Clinic for weekly wound care.

Although the right foot was ischaemic with a pressure index of 0.63, he was very careful to avoid injury and had no foot ulceration. Despite laser photocoagulation treatment his vision was very poor. The following year he suffered a cerebrovascular accident and became mute and wheelchair bound, but stayed at home, tended by his wife and children. Three months later his wife brought him to the Foot Clinic saying that he had a painful right first toe. There were no signs of cellulitis or swelling and the toe was not warm. Pedal pulses were absent. However, careful probing of the lateral sulcus of the right hallux elicited a discharge of pus (Figure 2.21) from a small abscess. A wound swab grew *Staphylococcus aureus* and Group B *Streptococcus*. This was a Stage 4 foot. The patient was admitted to hospital, in view of his frail condition and ischaemic status, and amoxycillin 500 mg tds and flucloxacillin 500 mg qds IV were prescribed. The foot healed quickly.

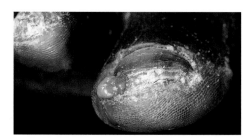

Figure 2.21   Probing of the lateral sulcus of the right hallux elicited a discharge of pus.

Learning points

- Acute ischaemia is a clinical emergency with severe morbidity and mortality. Revascularisation should be performed without delay and expert care of associated leg wounds from vein removal and grafting should be provided.

- Differential diagnosis between pain due to worsening ischaemia and pain due to infection can be difficult, especially where the skin is pigmented so that cellulitis is not obvious.

- It is dangerous to assume that worsening pain in an ischaemic foot is always due to worsening ischaemia. Infection should always be excluded and if there is any doubt about the diagnosis then antibiotics should also be given.

Case 2.22   Acute ischaemia – a clinical emergency

This case is a rare presentation of acute ischaemia in a diabetic patient.

A 64 year old lady with Type 2 diabetes of 17 years' duration was referred by telephone to the Foot Clinic by her general practitioner. The previous day she had developed pain and numbness in her left leg and was concerned that the colour of the foot was changing. She was seen the same day in the Foot Clinic. There was a temperature disparity of three degrees between the two feet. The left foot and lower leg were cold and painful, with a "cut-off" point at mid-calf where the temperature of the leg fell. Femoral pulses and the right popliteal and pedal pulses were present. Doppler studies revealed very little blood flow in the left foot and the colour of the toes was very poor (Figure 2.22).

In view of the discolouration of the toes, a Stage 5 foot was diagnosed, with acute ischaemia, and she was seen by the vascular surgeons and prepared for theatre the same day. Angiography revealed occlusion of superficial and popliteal arteries with good run-off at the ankle. A femoral to distal bypass was performed and restored pulsatile flow to the foot. Over the next three weeks the apices of the first, second, third and fourth toes developed dry necrosis, which was managed conservatively, gradually demarcated and autoamputated. Antibiotics were prescribed as required to control and eradicate infection and the foot healed in seven months. She had no further foot problems.

Learning points

- The majority of patients with neuroischaemic foot present as emergencies because of spreading infection.

- Less commonly patients present with acute ischaemia of the foot and leg, resulting from a sudden occlusion of the main leg arteries.

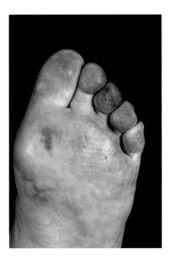

Figure 2.22   Dusky foot with blue discolouration of the toes.

- In non-diabetic patients without neuropathy this is extremely painful, but diabetic patients with neuroischaemic feet suffer less pain and this may delay their presentation.

- Acute ischaemia is a life-threatening condition. It is a clinical emergency and the patient must be taken to a hospital with an experienced vascular team without delay.

- Distal bypass can restore pulsatile flow to the foot and achieve rapid healing and is a cost effective treatment.

- This was a historic patient, treated in the early days of distal bypasses. VAC has now transformed the wound care management of these patients, and waiting for autoamputation of necrotic toes is now rarely done.

Case 2.23   Loss of two rays but healed after distal bypass

This patient was non-compliant but eventually responded to treatment and healed.

A 71 year old man with Type 2 diabetes of 9 years' duration was referred to the Diabetic Foot Clinic at King's as an emergency after he visited his general practitioner complaining of pain in the left foot and "blue toes". The foot was swollen and red, and the third and fourth toes were blue, with blue discolouration extending onto the dorsum of the forefoot (Figure 2.23a). The foot pulses were impalpable. Doppler studies revealed an ABPI of 1.86, but this was deemed to be artifactually high because of

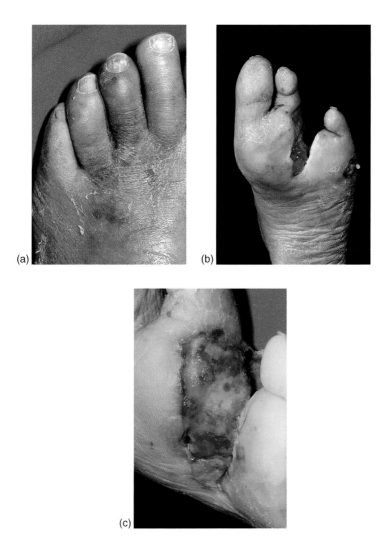

(a)   (b)   (c)

Figure 2.23 (a) Blue discolouration of the foot. (b) Ray amputation wound. (c) Split skin graft to wound.

arterial calcification. He was seen by the vascular team and underwent angiography, which revealed severe disease of the tibial vessels with good run-off at the ankle. This was a Stage 5 foot.

The surgeons performed amputation of the third and fourth rays and a distal bypass, following which the foot pulses could be palpated (Figure 2.23b). A split skin graft was applied to the wound (Figure 2.23c). A wide-fitting Dru-shoe with cushioned insole was provided. Oral antibiotics were prescribed, but he decided not to take them, and returned to the Foot Clinic one month later with infection of the ray amputation wound and ulceration over the plantar surface of the fifth metatarsal head. He then agreed to take antibiotics and the foot rapidly improved, although he had a subsequent admission for infection, which resulted in amputation of the fifth toe. A cradled insole was supplied to prevent further ulceration.

Learning points

- Arterial calcification leads to artifactual elevation of the ankle brachial pressure index because the sphygmomanometer cuff cannot compress the stiff vessels. For this reason, the ABPI reading should be taken in the clinical context. In this case, the foot looked ischaemic and the foot pulses were absent. In this context, a high ABPI was clearly inconsistent with the clinical picture.

- Following a successful distal bypass, previously ischaemic patients may develop plantar callus and ulceration over pressure points on the sole of the foot.

- Removal of two rays can lead to overloading of one or more adjoining rays, and a cradled insole may be needed to reduce plantar pressures.

2.5   Wound care

Neuroischaemic feet with large tissue defects need all the help they can get. Once infection control and revascularisation have been optimised there are other helpful techniques. Vacuum assisted wound closure is very useful. The VAC pump is used in two main scenarios. The most common of these is in the ischaemic foot after debridement when revascularisation has been performed. The second scenario is in ischaemic feet where revascularisation has not been possible. In these circumstances there is limited perfusion, but nevertheless a VAC pump can sometimes achieve healing.

Case 2.24   Post-operative wound care and successful use of VAC therapy on a large tissue defect

A 72 year old lady with Type 2 diabetes for 32 years and poor mobility lived on her own, with eight cats. She had hypertension, diabetic retinopathy, peripheral neuropathy and arterial disease. She was admitted via Casualty with a discoloured ischaemic left leg. On the medial aspect of her left foot was an infected, necrotic wound. This was a Stage 5 foot. She was confused and dehydrated. The CRP was 213.1 mg/l with a WBC of 19.45×10^9/l and neutrophils of 17.53×10^9/l, creatinine 262 µmol/l, and she was admitted to hospital and given IV fluids. She had had previous MRSA infections of the foot. She was prescribed IV vancomycin 1 g statim and then dosage according to serum levels, ceftazidime 1 g daily and metronidazole 500 mg tds. A wound swab grew mixed anaerobes and MRSA, and her antibiotics were focused down to vancomycin and metronidazole until the wound swabs were negative. She underwent vascular investigations, which revealed tibial disease. She underwent popliteal posterior tibial bypass, with amputation of the left first toe and debridement of surrounding non-viable tissue (Figure 2.24a). One day later she commenced VAC therapy. After four weeks of VAC therapy the wound improved (Figure 2.24b). The wound responded well (Figure 2.24c).

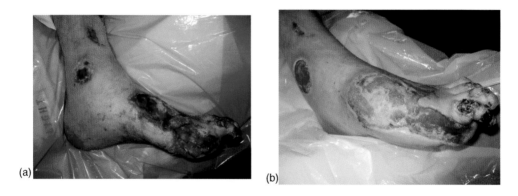

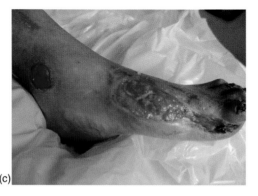

Figure 2.24 (a) Post-operative view of foot. (b) Granulation in the wound after 4 weeks' VAC therapy. (c) Healing wound after 8 weeks' VAC therapy.

Learning points

- Using VAC gives confidence to undertake minor amputations of ischaemic toes and to perform major debridements, even if revascularisation is not possible.

- VAC is useful in desloughing wounds that may have not been completely debrided.

- Wound care for the diabetic foot should involve regular wound inspections.

Case 2.25 VAC can sometimes achieve healing even if vascular intervention is not entirely successful

VAC was also used successfully on this patient even though revascularisation had not greatly improved perfusion of her neuroischaemic foot.

A lady with Type 2 diabetes, hypertension and neuroischaemic feet injured her left first toe, which developed infection and necrosis. She came to the Diabetic Foot Clinic with a Stage 5 foot. Her transcutaneous oxymetry was low at 34 mm Hg and she was admitted to hospital for an angiogram, which showed disease of the left superficial femoral, popliteal and tibial arteries. Angioplasty of superficial femoral and popliteal artery was successful (Figure 2.25a–c). However, although in the anterior tibial artery the proximal occlusion was opened using a 3 mm balloon, it was not possible to pass a wire through the distal occlusion, and a wire could not be passed through the peroneal artery. There was a reformation of the posterior tibial artery above the ankle to form part of the plantar arch.

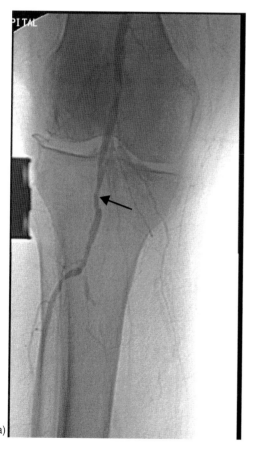
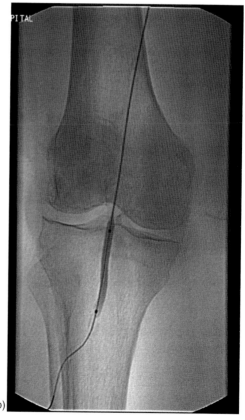

(a)   (b)

Figure 2.25 (a) Stenosis of the popliteal artery (arrow). (b) Ballooning of the popliteal artery stenosis.

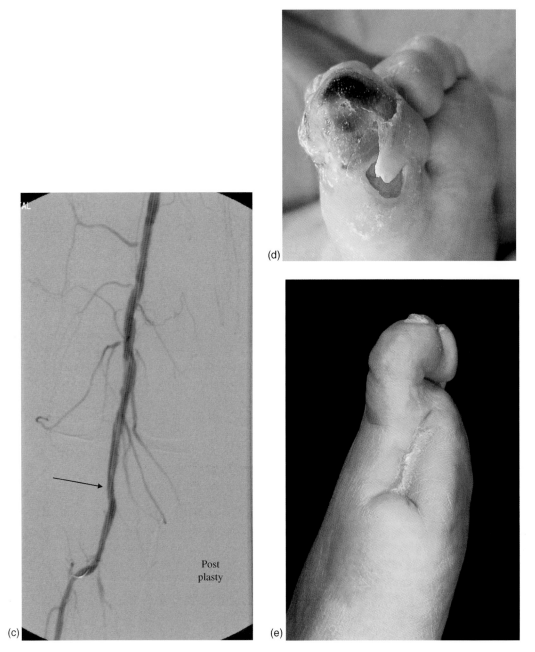

Figure 2.25 *(continued)* (c) Post angioplasty (arrow). (d) Necrotic toe. (e) Amputation site.

Her transcutaneous oxymetry remained low at 33 mm Hg. A wound swab of the first toe grew *Staphylococcus aureus* and *Stenotrophomonas maltophilia*, and she was treated with IV timentin 2.5 g tds. In view of the infection and necrosis (Figure 2.25d) her first toe was amputated (Figure 2.25e) and she then underwent VAC therapy. Although it had not been possible to achieve straight line flow, she healed with the VAC pump. She was followed in the Diabetic Foot Clinic

The following year she was admitted with an infected second toe on the right foot. X-ray showed soft tissue swelling and free gas within the soft tissues of the second toe, in keeping with infection. This was a Stage 4 foot. She was given IV amoxicillin 500 mg tds, flucloxacillin 500 mg qds, metronidazole 500 mg tds and ceftazidime 1 g tds. There was diffuse disease of the superficial femoral artery, diffuse narrowing of the popliteal artery and the peroneal and posterior tibial arteries were occluded, but the anterior tibial artery was patent with run-off to the foot, and angioplasty was performed to the popliteal with a 4 mm balloon with a good result. She had amputation of her second toe, and the wound healed without needing the VAC. *Staphylococcus aureus* was grown from the toe, and the antibiotics were focused to flucloxacillin.

Learning points

- In the early days of the Foot Clinic, in patients who developed digital necrosis, we sometimes faced a management dilemma: should we perform a minor amputation or should we treat the foot conservatively in the hope that the gangrenous toe would autoamputate? We would usually only remove the toe if it was possible to revascularise the patient.

- However, we will now often perform a minor amputation and use the VAC to achieve healing.

- This is especially the case when it is the first toe that becomes necrotic, as the results of autoamputation of this are poor.

2.6   Emboli

The next group of patients developed embolic lesions of the feet. It is always important to ascertain the source of the emboli.

Case 2.26   Popliteal aneurysm

A 78 year old man with Type 2 diabetes for 10 years had hypertension, ischaemic heart disease, schizophrenia and hypothyroidism, gout and depression. He had had a coronary artery bypass. One year later he developed claudication in both calves, which was worse on the right. He developed bilateral ulcers on the apices of toes associated with blueish discolouration of the surrounding skin. This was a Stage 3 foot. He was admitted for investigations and underwent MRA, which revealed bilateral popliteal artery aneurysms (Figure 2.26a). The aneurysm on the right had thrombosed completely, leading to popliteal occlusion. His angiogram showed very poor run-off, and none that could sustain a bypass graft. On the left side there was a patent popliteal aneurysm (Figure 2.26b). He was treated conservatively with aspirin and his ulcers slowly healed.

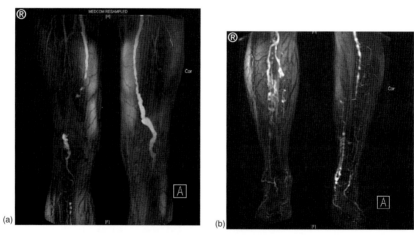

Figure 2.26   (a) Bilateral popliteal aneurysms with thrombosis on the right side. (b) Calf vessels on the right show no good run-off vessel although portions of the distal anterior tibial artery are seen. On the left no named run-off vessels are identified.

Learning points

- Diabetic patients with peripheral vascular disease may have popliteal artery aneurysms and they need a special approach.

- They differ from abdominal aortic aneurysms in one major respect in that they do not rupture but block off with thrombus, and this can lead to acute ischaemia of the leg, needing urgent bypass of the aneurysm.

- Thrombi formed in the aneurysm may throw off emboli that lodge lower down in the tibial vessels and foot arteries.

Case 2.27 Diffuse aortic plaque with thrombus

A 55 year old lady with diet controlled Type 2 diabetes diagnosed one year previously had undergone a coronary angiogram and stenting after she had a silent myocardial infarction. She presented to the Diabetic Foot Clinic with embolic lesions on the toes consisting of areas of discolouration and in particular a cold, painful, left second toe. This was a Stage 5 foot. She also had claudication in the left leg. An echocardiogram did not reveal a source of emboli from the left side of the heart. She had an angiogram performed, which showed narrowing at the level of the aortic bifurcation in the bilateral common iliac origins and also disease in the left proximal external iliac artery (Figure 2.27a). She therefore had a CT scan of the aorta, where a diffuse aortic plaque was found, with thrombus throughout the infra renal abdominal aorta (Figure 2.27b). An aortic endarterectomy was planned but was converted to an aorto-bifemoral bypass graft because of the very small calibre and heavy calcification of the aorta. The procedure improved her walking and she had no further embolic lesions. She was kept on aspirin and clopidogrel. The toe recovered. She remains on long term follow-up in the Diabetic Foot Clinic.

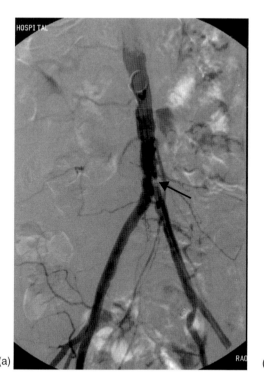

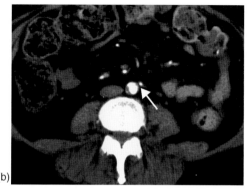

(a)   (b)

Figure 2.27 (a) Angiogram showing narrowing at the level of the aortic bifurcation (arrow) in the bilateral common iliac origins and also disease in the left proximal external iliac artery. (b) CT scan shows aortic plaque and thrombus (arrow).

Learning points

- When patients present with necrotic lesions of the toes, suggesting embolic lesions, it is important to search for the source of emboli, especially in the proximal arterial tree.

- Common sources of emboli are thrombus in the aortic and iliac arteries.

- The left atrium and ventricle of the heart can also be a source of emboli.

- Silent myocardial infarcts may occur in diabetic patients. The patient who looks awful, pale, sweaty and clammy may be having an myocardial infarction although he does not have chest pain.

Case 2.28   Good pulses, black necrotic toe

This 75 year old man had hypertension and Type 2 diabetes of 20 years' duration. He had diabetic nephropathy and also had an IgA nephropathy. He presented with shortness of breath and acute left ventricular failure, cardiogenic shock, acute myocardial infarction and an episode of ventricular tachycardia, and a coronary angiogram showed severe triple vessel coronary artery disease. A coronary artery bypass was performed. He also had a right renal artery stenosis, which had a stent insertion.

He presented six months later at the Diabetic Foot Clinic with a necrotic left fourth toe tip and palpable pedal pulses. This was a Stage 5 foot (Figure 2.28a). Creatinine was 200 μmol/l, and eGFR was 32 ml/min. He grew *Staphylococcus aureus*, *Pseudomonas aeruginosa* and anaerobic *Streptococcus*. Antibiotics were prescribed orally, namely flucloxacillin 500 mg qds, ciprofloxacin 500 mg bd and metronidazole 400 mg tds. The lesion was thought to be embolic and he had a Duplex angiography of the aorta, which revealed an aortic aneurysm of 3 cm diameter with thrombus. This was asymptomatic. A CT scan with IV contrast was performed with IV fluids and N-acetylcysteine 600 mg bd for 24 hours before and after the scan. This confirmed an infra-renal aortic aneurysm measuring 4.1 cm × 0.6 cm. The iliac vessels were ectatic. There were two small internal iliac aneurysms, 1.3 cm on the left and 1.6 cm on the right (Figure 2.28b). He was anticoagulated with warfarin and aspirin. The necrotic toe tip shelled off. He has regular surveillance of the aneurysms and follow-up in the Diabetic Foot Clinic.

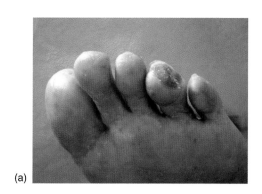
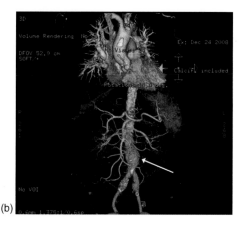

(a) (b)

Figure 2.28   (a) Necrotic 4th toe. (b) Aortic aneurysm, shown on CT angiogram (arrow).

Learning points

- In a foot with good pedal pulses and black toe, the differential diagnosis includes infection or embolus.

- If embolus is diagnosed a search should be made for the source.

- Duplex angiography is a useful initial investigation. If an aortic aneurysm is suspected, then a CT scan with contrast should be carried out.

- If renal function is impaired, then a CT scan should be performed with N-acetylcysteine cover as well as with IV fluids.

2.7 Complications

2.7.1 Complications post angioplasty

The next section of this chapter presents cases of complications following revascularisation, beginning with angioplasty. We do not want to give the impression that complication rates are high, but to share the lessons we have learned from the very occasional complications encountered in our patients.

Angioplasty is usually a very safe technique, and we would like to emphasise this point. So widely used is angioplasty that it is usually performed on a day case basis and the only patients needing admission for the procedure are those who are very frail, for example patients with severe renal impairment. Angioplasty is a very useful technique but we have sometimes seen complications, which are described in some of the case studies below. We include a patient with a haemorrhagic scrotum following angioplasty, and the next case, a lady who serves as a warning to all practitioners of the dangers of a retroperitoneal bleed in patients with concomitant neuropathy, who do not show the classical signs of fluid loss, and may even fail to put up their pulse in response when their blood pressure drops.

Case 2.29   Retroperitoneal bleed following angioplasty

A 68 year old lady with Type 2 diabetes of 16 years' duration, peripheral neuropathy with a VPT of 40 V, peripheral vascular disease and cerebrovascular accident resulting in left hemiplegia developed a pressure sore over her left lateral malleolus (Figure 2.29a) and was referred to the Diabetic Foot Clinic. This was a Stage 3 foot. She lived at home with her husband and the district nurses called every day. She was given a Dru shoe, cut away at

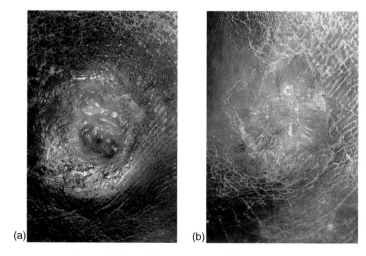

(a)   (b)

Figure 2.29   (a) Pressure sore. (b) Healed ulcer.

the ankle to avoid any pressure on the ulcer, which was dressed every day with a foam dressing and light bandage. The ulcer healed in 14 weeks (Figure 2.29b).

She had a relapse of ulceration on the same site when she stopped wearing the Dru shoe, but when this was reinstated the ulcer healed in three weeks. She did well for three more years but then developed ischaemic ulceration on the apices of her left toes and the third toe became gangrenous. The foot became painful. This was now a Stage 5 foot. She underwent angiography, and suffered a retroperitoneal bleed. She felt no pain and her pulse rate did not increase: in fact, the only sign that anything was wrong was that she dropped her blood pressure two hours post procedure. She underwent fluid resuscitation and an emergency laparotomy to repair an iliac artery perforation.

As regards her foot, she was treated conservatively with liberal analgesia, reduction of oedema, regular cleansing and dressing of the ulcer and systemic antibiotics. She died of a cerebrovascular accident the following year. This happened in the days before VAC was available.

Learning points

- This case occurred in the early days of the Diabetic Foot Clinic. Such retroperitoneal bleeds are nowadays almost unknown with the use of small bore arterial cannulae.

- A fall in blood pressure post angiography should be investigated and treated immediately.

- If diabetic foot patients do bleed, they may not develop a tachycardia because of their co-existent neuropathy.

- Many patients with ischaemic ulcers respond well to conservative care.

- Footwear should be adapted to offload pressure where necessary.

Case 2.30   Plaque dislodged during angioplasty leads to gangrene of the toes

One of the commonest complications of angioplasty arises when thrombus or plaque is dislodged and travels distally to the feet.

A 76 year old lady with Type 1 diabetes of 59 years' duration, diabetic nephropathy and proliferative retinopathy treated with laser photocoagulation, autonomic neuropathy with history of gustatory sweating and diabetic diarrhoea, and peripheral sensory neuropathy with VPT of 32 V, was referred to the Diabetic Foot Clinic complaining of rest pain affecting the left foot. There was no tissue defect and a Stage 2 foot was diagnosed. The ABPI was 0.47 and she complained of intermittent claudication at a distance of 20 yards. She was admitted for angiography and a tight stenosis of the superficial femoral artery was dilated.

Six hours later, although pulsatile flow had been restored to the foot, it was noticed that the apices of the first, third and fifth toes had developed blue discolouration and they became necrotic. This was now a Stage 5 foot, it being thought that debris had been released from a proximal arterial plaque during angioplasty. The discoloured areas became necrotic. She was offered conservative care with antibiotics, regular debridement and wide fitting shoes. The worst affected toe was the fifth, which was frankly necrotic.

Within six weeks this toe autoamputated and the apices of the first and third toes shed necrotic material and healed.

Learning points

- Angioplasty is usually safe but is not entirely without complications. If plaque is disturbed and breaks loose to travel distally then it can occlude digital vessels, leading to local ischaemia and necrosis.

- Thrombolysis should be commenced without delay if thrombus is dislodged.

- Long-term outcomes can be good if the ischaemic status of the foot has been improved by the angioplasty.

2.7.2   Complications post bypass

Most of the complications following arterial bypass are related to existing co-morbidities of diabetic ischaemic patients or to the development of intercurrent infections.

Case 2.31 Bypass patient who developed *C. difficile* infection

This patient with diabetes and hyperlipidaemia also had a history of ulcerative colitis, for which he took mesalazine 400 mg tds, and primary pan sclerosing cholangitis and cirrhosis. He had previously undergone an elective coronary artery graft bypass × 3 in September 2001. He had claudication at ten yards with rest pain and developed an ulcer on the left foot. He presented at the Diabetic Foot Clinic with an ischaemic ulcer of the left foot. This was a Stage 3 foot. His MRA showed moderate narrowing of the left common iliac artery and occlusion of the left superficial femoral artery. He underwent balloon dilatation of the left common iliac artery to 8 mm (Figure 2.31a, b). He underwent a left femoral popliteal bypass.

Post-operatively, he developed diarrhoea. This condition was associated with a very high WBC of 30.00×10^9/l and a neutrophilia of 26.00×10^9/l. His WBC rose to 39.28×10^9/l, with a CRP of 182.8 mg/l. His creatinine rose from 102 to 243 μmol/l, falling again to 113 μmol/l on the sixth post-operative day. The faecal specimen grew *Clostridium difficile*. On examination, he had a mildly tender abdomen with slight distension. The chest was clear and the leg wounds were not infected. He had previously been on amoxicillin for a Group G *Streptococcus* isolated from his foot. This man had multiple co-morbidities and may have been predisposed to *C. difficile* by pre-existing ulcerative colitis. He was treated with metronidazole 400 mg tds and made a full recovery.

Learning points

- One of the most unpleasant complications of antibiotic therapy is infection of the gastrointestinal tract with *C. difficile* following use of antibiotics.

- We have seen very few patients who have developed *C. difficile* infection, but clinicians need to be aware of the signs and symptoms. There are some particularly virulent strains

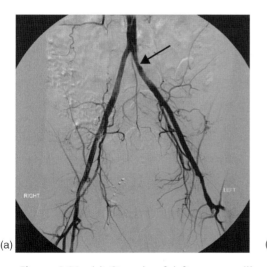
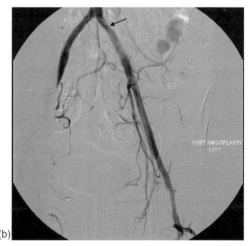

(a) (b)

Figure 2.31 (a) Stenosis of left common iliac artery (arrow). (b) Post angioplasty. Stenosis dilated (arrow)

of *C. difficile* (E21), which produce more toxin, and some hospitals have had high mortality rates.

- It is necessary to have a high index of suspicion, and send stool specimens to confirm the diagnosis. A high white count (around 30.00×10^9/l) is typical of a *C. difficile* infection.

- We treat initially with metronidazole orally; if there is no response we then change to vancomycin 125 mg qds, given orally.

- In severe cases, practitioners must be aware of the development of a pan colitis. A CT scan may be helpful in diagnosis, showing colonic wall thickening, and the patient may need a total colectomy to save his life.

- This was not needed in this patient, because, for us, diarrhoea in a diabetic patient treated with antibiotics always rings the alarm bells and we assume a worst case scenario, which is always wise when managing the diabetic foot.

- Diabetic patients with neuropathy will not have classical signs and symptoms. Although this patient had a marked *C. difficile* infection, he did not have significant abdominal discomfort and he was only mildly tender on examination. This lack of discomfort may have been related to his neuropathy.

Case 2.32 Dialysis after bypass

This patient developed infection following a bypass, and needed dialysis.

A 70 year old man had Type 2 diabetes of 37 years' duration treated with insulin. He had a coronary artery bypass graft and hypertension, and his serum creatinine was 140 μmol/l. He was seen at the Diabetic Foot Clinic with a necrotic right third toe (Figure 2.32). This was a Stage 5 foot. The necrosis was dry with no signs of infection. He was admitted to hospital. A Duplex scan showed no stenosis of the femoral and popliteal arteries. The necrotic right third toe was amputated. The wound became sloughy and he was given quadruple antibiotics, amoxicillin 500 mg tds, flucloxacillin 500 mg qds, metronidazole 500 mg tds and ceftazidime 1 g tds, which were narrowed down to flucloxacillin when *Staphylococcus aureus* was grown from a wound swab. He was discharged to be followed up in the Diabetic Foot Clinic.

Two months later, it was noted that his creatinine had risen to 200 μmol/l with eGFR of 30 ml/min. He had a *Klebsiella pneumoniae* infection of the right third toe stump, which was treated with IM imipenem 500 mg bd. A further two months on, his right third toe amputation site became infected and he developed a sloughy ulcer on his right first toe. This was a Stage 4 foot. Wound swabs grew *Staphylococcus aureus* and *Klebsiella pneumoniae*, which were treated with flucloxacillin and imipenem.

After a further 3 months, the right first toe was very ischaemic and he underwent angiography and attempted angioplasty but a distal posterior tibial occlusion could not be crossed. A distal arterial bypass was then attempted but no run-off artery could be found at operation. His creatinine was now 220 μmol/l and his eGFR was 27 ml/min.

He recovered well, but developed diarrhoea from a norovirus infection and his creatinine rose to 259 μmol/l. Next day it was 380 μmol/l, and the following day it had risen to 511 μmol/l, with a WBC of 14.04×10^9/l, of which neutrophils were 12.03×10^9/l. He was dialysed in the early hours of the next day and his creatinine came down

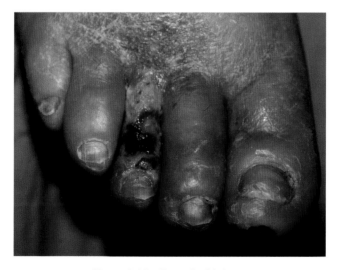

Figure 2.32 Necrotic third toe.

to 392 µmol/l. He was positive for *Norovirus* Genogroup 2RNA in the faeces but *Clostridium difficile* toxin was not detected. He also had a urinary tract infection with more than 100, 000 orgs per ml of *Klebsiella* species from a catheter specimen. He was treated with gentamicin. He was eventually able to come off dialysis.

Learning points

- Episodes of recurrent sepsis in the foot damaged this man's renal function.

- Eventually, two serious systemic postoperative infections caused severe impairment of renal function such that dialysis was needed.

- When diarrhoea develops in diabetic foot patients, it is important to send faeces urgently for microbiological investigations including *Clostridium difficile* and norovirus infections

- Moreover, urinary tract infections are so frequent in diabetic patients that it is always wise to send urine for microbiological investigations.

- As illustrated in this case, diabetic patients are supremely vulnerable to infection.

2.8 Pain in the neuroischaemic foot

Pain is rarely present in the diabetic neuroischaemic foot because of the presence of neuropathy; however, when the patient complains of pain the most likely causes are ischaemic rest pain, infection or painful neuropathy.

Case 2.33 The ischaemic patient with pain: is it rest pain or neuropathic pain?

This 65 year old man was a recently diagnosed Type 2 diabetic patient who complained of burning pain in both legs at rest of increasing severity. He also had decreasing exercise tolerance. Previously a Duplex scan had shown that he had severe bilateral iliac artery stenosis as well as distal disease in the superficial femoral artery with occlusion of the popliteal on the right. Bilateral iliac stents were inserted but the left big toe subsequently became dusky. This was a Stage 2 foot. He was readmitted for angioplasty and started on warfarin. The patient underwent bilateral superficial femoral artery/popliteal artery angioplasty. He took tramadol 50 mg qds for pain together with aspirin 150 mg od and his feet improved.

After the endoluminal intervention, he had some residual burning pains across both feet and in his toes but his symptoms were less and he was able to walk 200–300 yards prior to getting calf claudication. He was started on gabapentin and amitriptyline for his neuropathic pain. Five months later he had an ABPI of 0.62 on the right and 0.55 on the left but there were significant drops of ABPI with exercise.

Eight weeks after this, he had increasing pain in the left foot and leg. He also had superficial ulcers on the left foot, which was now a Stage 3 foot. The Duplex angiogram showed that the stents were functioning well in his iliacs. On the left he had stenosis at the origin of the profunda femoris artery, together with multiple stenoses along the superficial femoral artery and disease extending beyond this down to the ankle. He had left superficial femoral artery and popliteal artery angioplasty four weeks later and the rest pain significantly improved. The dorsalis pedis artery returned on the left side and was palpable post angioplasty, which is rare.

He then complained of right-sided pain. He developed an ulcer on the right third metatarsal head with a dry, gangrenous patch over the hallux (Stage 5 foot), which responded to conservative therapy. After five months, he complained of intermittent claudication in the calf and buttocks and Duplex showed a tight common femoral artery stenosis on the right side and a superficial femoral artery stenosis on the left side. He was treated conservatively.

Learning points

- It is difficult to separate neuropathic pain from ischaemic pain. They are both present at rest. Classically, the neuropathic pain has a more burning quality. This patient had bilateral pain, worse at rest, aggravated by wearing clothes but relieved by putting the foot out of bed at night.

- He had angiography, which showed definite evidence of peripheral arterial disease. Arterial stenosis and occlusions were angioplastied and stented, which partially relieved his pain but did not completely relieve it.

- When ischaemic patients present with pain, it is important first to relieve arterial stenoses and occlusions. If the pain persists, then it may have an important neuropathic element, which should be treated with appropriate anticonvulsants or tricyclic antidepressant medication.

2.9 Conservative care

This section is to emphasise the importance of conservative care. It includes some historical cases taken from the 1980s, when revascularisation was not possible. Nevertheless, it does indicate what can be achieved with conservative care, and this is important in the modern day if such technologies are not available or the patient declines active intervention. However, we feel that almost any diabetic patient can be put forward for angioplasty, as the only requirement is to be able to lie flat for 30 minutes and undertake a local anaesthetic procedure.

Case 2.34   Tender loving care at home

This 70 year old diabetic lady with Type 2 diabetes for 10 years had multiple comorbidities, and an ulcer of the left foot and leg, which became infected by MRSA. She had extensive cerebrovascular disease with left hemiparesis from stroke, hypertension, bilateral cataracts and a coronary artery bypass graft. She was immobile, and lived at home with her daughter. The anterior tibial ulcer, also involving the dorsum of the foot, developed extensive necrosis. This was a Stage 5 foot. She had previously undergone vascular assessment and was deemed not to be angioplastable.

She was admitted and treated with IV vancomycin 1 g statim and then dosage according to serum levels. This controlled infection and the necrosis stopped spreading. A CT scan of the head showed old extensive infarction with no new areas of haemorrhage but the previous infarctions had involved the left cerebellar hemisphere and the right middle cerebral artery.

She underwent recurrent admissions, but hated coming into hospital, and her daughter wanted her mother "to die at home". On her last admission a chest X-ray showed peri hilar air space shadowing and patchy consolidation at the left base indicative of pneumonia. She received palliative care and eventually died.

Learning points

- Ischaemic necrosis in the diabetic foot is frequently complicated by sepsis, and some patients respond well to treatment with antibiotics.

- Diabetic ischaemic patients have multiple comorbidities. In some cases, they become overwhelming and it is apparent that the patient only has a few days or weeks to live.

- The transition to this phase in the natural history of diabetes must be recognised and the appropriate palliative care carried out.

- The wishes of patients and family members regarding admission and treatment should always be respected.

Case 2.35   Autoamputation of an ischaemic gangrenous toe

This case is another historic one from the King's archive, from the days before VAC was available, where we attempted to achieve healing of a black toe by conservative means when no angioplasty or reconstruction was possible.

A 76 year old Afro-Caribbean woman with Type 2 diabetes of 9 years' duration treated with diet alone was aware of pain and throbbing in her right second toe and visited her general practitioner, who sent her to see the practice nurse. She realised that the toe was infected and necrotic and telephoned the Diabetic Foot Clinic, and the patient was seen the same afternoon. She had a Stage 5 foot. There was a VPT of 40 V. Pedal pulses in the left foot were weak and those in the right foot were absent. Transcutaneous oxymetry was 25 mm Hg. She was admitted and underwent angiography but there was no angioplastable or reconstructable vascular lesion.

Tissue from the toe grew *Escherichia coli* and mixed anaerobes. Intravenous ceftazidime 1 g tds and metronidazole 500 mg tds were prescribed and the necrosis became dry and well demarcated. Because vascular intervention was not feasible it was decided to treat her conservatively with a view to achieving autoamputation of the necrotic toe. Good control of her diabetes was achieved with insulin. A diuretic was prescribed to reduce oedema, and on discharge after two weeks she was given oral antibiotics. The district nurses visited her every day. The foot was kept clean and dry with dressings inserted between the toes to prevent contact between the gangrenous toe and its neighbours. No surgical tape was applied to the foot: instead the dressings were held in place with a light bandage. She came to the Foot Clinic every two weeks for debridement along the demarcation line between gangrene and viable tissue, and after seven months the toe dropped off and the foot healed.

Learning points

- Patients who have gangrene and are not suitable for revascularisation will sometimes respond well to conservative care and major amputation is not inevitable.

- Successful autoamputation demands meticulous foot care from a dedicated team.

- After complete healing has occurred the patient should be followed up in the foot clinic.

Case 2.36 To amputate or not... that is the question

This man was a very frail ischaemic patient, aged 73. Two years previously he had suffered two strokes. He had a right hemiparesis with contractures of the leg and was mute. His Type 2 diabetes was of 20 years' duration, and he had retinopathy and hypertension. There was widespread ulceration of the right foot, and he was admitted for angiography and right popliteal stenoses were dilated. He was readmitted four weeks later and stayed in hospital until he died. In view of his previous strokes and his right hemiparesis he was not a candidate for arterial bypass. He developed widespread necrosis and severe pain and entered Stage 6. He underwent a right above the knee amputation.

Initially, he made a good recovery but then became septic, from uncertain cause, but *Pseudomonas* was isolated from his Hickman line, and he was started on piperacillin–tazobactam 4.5 g tds. He then developed rest pain in the remaining foot and underwent angiography with dilatation of the left popliteal artery. He was relatively stable for one month and his rest pain was relieved, but he was unable to get out of bed. He then had two episodes of coffee ground vomitus, and collapsed and died. Post mortem showed acute myocardial infarction, with pulmonary congestion with oedema. Gastric mucosa was normal. The brain showed two old infarcts, one in the left frontal lobe and one in the left parietal lobe. He had not complained of chest pain.

Learning points

- When patients have very severe rest pain which cannot be controlled with liberal analgesia and cannot be revascularised, such patients should come to major amputation sooner rather than later.

- However, it should never be forgotten that pain in the ischaemic foot is not always due to ischaemia: look for infection, which is a common cause of pain in the neuroischaemic foot.

- When the right foot of this patient developed severe pain and necrosis, it was difficult to decide whether the patient should have a major amputation or receive palliative therapy. What would the reader have advised?

- In the event, a major amputation was carried out. Although the patient survived the operation, his remaining weeks of life were not happy ones.

3
Charcot Case Studies

3.1 Introduction

Charcot's osteoarthropathy is one of the most mysterious, challenging and interesting complications of the diabetic foot. It can develop without apparent cause, though careful questioning will usually elicit a history of an insult, which may be a sprain or a fall, walking on uneven surfaces such as cobblestones or rapid remobilisation after a period of non-weight-bearing in a bed. It is our impression that any event leading to hyperaemia in a foot – including infection – can trigger a Charcot joint. However, it is fascinating that the same patient may have previously undergone a similar episode of hyperaemia without initiating the Charcot process.

Almost without exception our Charcot patients have small fibre neuropathy (many have large fibre neuropathy too), autonomic neuropathy and a good blood supply to the feet: we have only seen two cases of patients who developed Charcot's osteoarthropathy in an ischaemic foot, and both are described in this chapter. The patients with Type 1 diabetes have osteoporosis in their feet before the Charcot develops and usually first present with fractures: the Type 2 patients do not have osteoporosis prior to the development of the Charcot and are more likely to present with subluxation and dislocation.

When the Diabetic Foot Clinic at King's started up in the early 1980s the patients with Charcot feet were seen by the orthopaedic surgeon, and were encouraged to rest as much as possible and to offload the foot with crutches. If they presented with an obvious fracture then they were put into conventional below-knee walking casts, as for simple fractures. We even saw cases of patients who had been seen in the Casualty departments of other hospitals and told that they did not need a cast because the foot was not painful. We have also seen patients with diabetes and a fracture who were taken out of a cast after six weeks without the foot being re-X-rayed to ensure that healing of the fracture was adequate (in our experience it takes at least twice as long to heal a fracture in a diabetic foot as in a non-diabetic foot). Furthermore, we have learned that if the patient is caught early the X-ray will be normal, but a bone scan, MRI or CT scan will detect early changes.

Many of the early Charcot patients developed severe deformity and instability. They were given surgical shoes or boots to accommodate the deformity: some used old-fashioned leg irons, crutches or wheelchairs. It was difficult to persuade patients who felt

Diabetic Foot Care: Case Studies in Clinical Management   Alethea Foster and Michael Edmonds
© 2011 John Wiley & Sons, Ltd.

no pain to comply with treatment. Then, in 1987 the authors visited the Carville Institute, at Baton Rouge, Louisiana, USA, a state-funded leprosy hospital where Dr. Paul Brand's team used the total contact cast to treat people with leprosy who had neuropathic ulcers or Charcot joints. We learned the casting technique there and brought it back to the United Kingdom, where it continues to play a major part in our management of the complicated neuropathic foot with indolent ulcers or acute Charcot. We have adapted the original Paul Brand technique to incorporate extra cast padding to minimise iatrogenic lesions, and one of the authors was interested, on a recent visit to Karigiri, where Brand first casted Indian patients, to find that there too the original Brand technique has been changed in the same way. We have been running casting courses for many years so that other practitioners can be taught this gold-standard treatment. We sometimes use an Aircast for patients who are awaiting a bone scan to confirm the diagnosis, and for people who cannot or will not use a total contact cast. For rehabilitation we use special footwear, the Charcot Restraint Orthotic Walker (CROW) and the ankle–foot orthosis.

Another major change over the 29 years that the King's Foot Clinic has been running has been in the approach to surgery for the patient with a deformed Charcot foot. In the early years of the Clinic the only operations ever performed were an exostectomy to shave bone off protruding plantar prominences in rocker-bottom feet, or drainage and debridement of acute infections. It was known that attempts to operate on acute Charcot feet in order to correct deformity or instability led to disaster, with screws and plates working loose and new fractures and dislocations developing – almost as if the surgery were exacerbating the Charcot process.

Recently, indications for surgery, which include acute dislocation, recurrent ulceration and unstable deformity, and the optimal timing of the procedure have been explored. The important thing is to wait until the acute stage is over and the redness, warmth and swelling have resolved, as surgery performed during the acute phase will indeed exacerbate the Charcot. However, once the foot has cooled down it is then safe to operate, and some very complicated procedures are now undertaken: sometimes including the use of the Taylor Spatial Frame, which uses computerised software to achieve correction of deformity along several different planes, after which the foot may be stabilised with rods or plates. Long and careful rehabilitation is always needed, since if the patient walks too early the operation will not be successful.

Use of these techniques has illustrated once again how very frail and vulnerable the high-risk diabetic foot patient is. Some of these Charcot patients appear very robust and active and they are anxious to lead as normal a life as they possibly can. While using the Taylor Spatial Frame to correct severe deformity in patients with Charcot's osteoarthropathy is an exciting development, it is our experience that diabetic Charcot patients treated with the Taylor Spatial Frame have sometimes had problems with infected pins or broken pins. Patients with neuropathy, impaired vision, lack of protective pain sensation, poor proprioception, hypotension and high body mass index tend to be very prone to infection and also to be clumsy, and they are very liable to damage their frames. (We have seen similar problem in patients using Aircasts also: one of our patients probably holds the world record for damaging seven Aircasts in the course of six weeks, and another fell and broke his leg in an Aircast.)

Although the outcomes of modern surgical techniques are good, Charcot deformity should be prevented so that surgery can be avoided if possible, since in people with diabetes the complications of surgery are more likely. Moreover, people with Charcot's osteoarthropathy are very prone to develop the perioperative complications already described in the section on neuropathy.

Without rapid active treatment the Charcot process can destroy the normal architecture of the foot or ankle very quickly, leading to severe deformity, instability and ulceration. We believe that the key to success is to keep these patients free of deformity. If their diabetic lives are long, they will often develop peripheral vascular disease, and go from having a neuropathic Charcot foot to a neuroischaemic Charcot foot, with ischaemia superimposed years after the Charcot foot first developed. Patients often get away with foot deformity while they are neuropaths, but once they develop ischaemia it is difficult to get any ulcers healed if the foot is deformed. The gold-standard treatment for the Charcot joint is the total contact cast, and successful management and prevention of deformity and instability depends upon catching the problem early. Good long-term follow-up is also important. However, even if the patient develops deformity or instability, this can often be managed with good footwear and orthotics, or even surgery. We never give up. The CROW or even a PTBWRO can salvage the end stage Charcot foot.

In this section we include case histories illustrating different presentations of Charcot, in different sites, complicated or uncomplicated. Some of the cases demonstrate that if a Charcot foot is caught early and treated in a suitable cast, then deformity can be prevented. We also describe some unfortunate patients who are very prone to fractures and Charcots, with multiple episodes. And we finish with some historic cases of patients who coped long term with conservative management.

The sections of this chapter are as follows:

- Early diagnosis

- Different presentations
  Type 1 patients with osteopaenia
  Infections in the Charcot foot
  Gout and the Charcot foot
  The neuroischaemic Charcot foot

- Surgery
  Internal fixation
  External fixation
  Exostectomy

- Conservative care.

At this stage we would like to pay tribute to our consultant orthopaedic surgeons for their skilful reconstruction of Charcot feet, including Venu Kavarthapu, Om Lahoti, Graeme Groom, Sara Phillips and Mark Phillips. Also at this juncture we would like to thank David Elias, Consultant Radiologist, for his very helpful interpretation of MRIs and CT scans of Charcot feet and Muriel Buxton-Thomas, Mazin AM Al-Janabi Nicola Mulholland and Gill Vivian also for very helpful interpretation of nuclear medicine scans.

3.2 Early diagnosis

Case 3.1   Avoiding deformity in Charcot feet

This lady had episodes of Charcot ostoearthropathy, which were caught early and treated actively: she did not develop deformity.

She was 64 years old, with Type 1 diabetes of 41 years' duration. She had proliferative retinopathy, which was treated with pan retinal photocoagulation. She developed her first Charcot foot after she had been to her local hospital as an emergency after a fall, and they found a fracture of the base of the fifth metatarsal of her left foot. She was casted for a conventional period of two weeks, following which the cast was removed without a further X-ray. She had notified the Foot Clinic about her accident and we asked her to come and see us as soon as the cast was removed. She came to the Diabetic Foot Clinic the same day, and we re-X-rayed the foot and found an unhealed fracture. This was a Stage 2 foot. We put her in a cast, where she remained for many months. By 14 months, the fracture was healing and by 16 months there was evidence of bony union. She was fully rehabilitated after two years.

Six years later, she had a second episode of Charcot. She presented with swelling over the dorsum of the right foot. X-ray was normal (Figure 3.1a), but a technetium diphosphonate bone scan showed greatly increased uptake over the right mid-foot (Figure 3.1b). A removable bivalved cast was applied. An MRI of the right mid-foot showed prominent marrow oedema at the base of the second metatarsal and also within the middle cuneiform (Figure 3.1c). On the sagittal image (Figure 3.1d) there was an intra-articular non-displaced fracture at the plantar aspect of the base of the second metatarsal. The Lisfranc ligament was reported to be thickened and irregular at its attachment to the second metatarsal, but there was no malalignment. A total contact cast was applied. She had a follow-up MRI six months later, when the marrow oedema within the second metatarsal and the middle cuneiform had virtually resolved (Figure 3.1e). The fracture line at the base of the second metatarsal was still just apparent, but was consistent with a healed previous fracture. The mid-foot remained correctly aligned. The Lisfranc ligament was noted to be abnormal, with irregularity, oedema and enhancement across it. X-ray at this time showed patchy osteopaenia and sclerosis. Three months later, she moved to an Aircast from a total contact cast, as the foot temperatures were within 2 °C. Despite her bilateral Charcot feet, she had no specific deformity or ulceration.

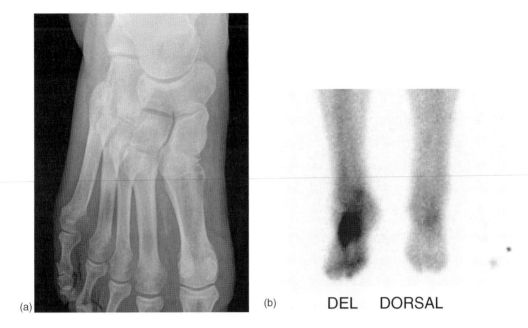

(a)

(b)   DEL   DORSAL

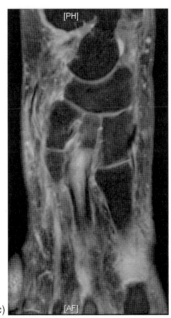

(c)

Figure 3.1   (a) Normal X-ray in early Charcot. (b) Greatly increased uptake over right mid-foot is seen on bone scan. DEL = delayed phase (c) MRI showing STIR sequence. Prominent marrow oedema at the base of the second metatarsal and also within the middle cuneiform.

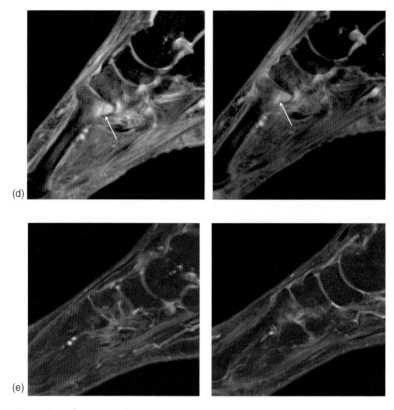

Figure 3.1 (*continued*) (d) MRI showing STIR sequence (left) and post gadolinium sequence (right). Intra-articular non-displaced fracture at the plantar aspect of the base of the second metatarsal (arrows). (e) MRI showing STIR sequence (left) and postgadolinium sequence (right). Resolution of marrow oedema.

Learning points

- Even though the X-ray may be normal, early diagnosis can be made by noting increased uptake on the technetium diphosphonate bone scan and bone marrow oedema on the MRI.

- If the Charcot foot is caught early and casted it can heal with good alignment.

- Fractures take much longer to heal in people with diabetes compared with non-diabetic patients.

- Re-X-ray to check healing in people with diabetes who have fractures should be mandatory before casts are removed.

Case 3.2   Early diagnosis

Even if the Charcot joint is caught early, management can be very challenging, especially when there are severe concurrent comorbidities.

This 45 year old lady with Type 1 diabetes for 21 years had diabetic retinopathy and postural hypotension together with gastroparesis. She had also undergone renal transplantation. She had osteopaenia and recurrent urinary tract infection. She had severe widespread autonomic neuropathy affecting her cardiovascular function. She presented with swelling of the left foot. X-ray (Figure 3.2a) was normal but the technetium diphosphonate bone scan showed increased uptake in the talonavicular region (Figure 3.2b). MRI showed oedema of the proximal talus and the navicular (Figure 3.2c) and she was treated in a total contact cast. The Charcot foot with unbroken skin is a Stage 2 foot and she fell into this category. When the final total contact cast was removed, the foot remained free from deformity and MRI showed resolution of the oedema of the distal talus and the navicular (Figure 3.2d).

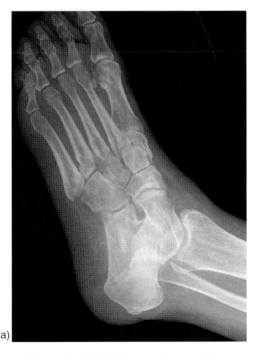

(a)

Figure 3.2   (a) Early X-ray is normal.

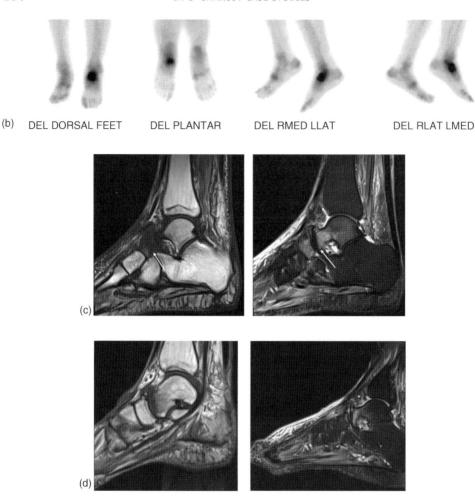

Figure 3.2 (*continued*) (b) Bone scan shows increased uptake at talonavicular region. DEL = delayed phase, Dorsal, Plantar, Medial and Lateral views (c) MRI showing T1 sequence (left) and STIR sequence (right) with oedema of talus and navicular (arrows). (d) MRI showing T1 sequence (left) and STIR sequence (right) with resolution of the oedema of talus and navicular.

Learning points

- This patient demonstrates the development of a Charcot foot in the background of severe, complicated Type 1 diabetes. The patient had multiple complications, namely retinopathy, neuropathy and nephropathy. The patient had underlying osteopaenia.

- A swollen, hot foot in a diabetic patient, especially with autonomic neuropathy, should be treated as a Charcot foot until proven otherwise.

- Renal transplant patients are particularly prone to develop Charcot joints.

- In the context of the patient's presentation, bone marrow oedema is diagnostic of Charcot foot.

Case 3.3   Normal X-ray, with abnormal bone scan and abnormal MRI

This case was caught very early, before there were X-ray changes in his Charcot foot.

A 58 year old man with Type 1 diabetes for 24 years fell and developed a hot swollen left foot. He was sent for an X-ray, which was normal, and reported no fractures and no dislocations. The left foot was over 3 °C hotter than the right foot, so he was treated with an Aircast while a technetium diphosphonate bone scan was arranged. This showed hotspots of increased uptake in the mid and hind foot. He then had a MRI (Figure 3.3a), which showed marrow oedema and enhancement within the mid cuboid and there was a linear horizontal line within the cuboid on the T1 weighted images consistent with trabecular microfracture. There was also oedema within the bases of the second and third metatarsals and within the middle and lateral cuneiforms.

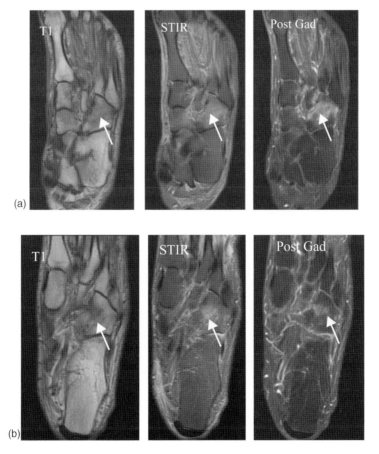

Figure 3.3   (a) MRI at presentation with T1, STIR and post-gadolinium sequences showing marrow oedema in mid foot and trabecular microfracture of the cuboid (arrows). (b) MRI at 3 months with reduction in oedema, particularly in the navicular, cuneiforms and second and third metatarsal bases. There remains some oedema through the cuboid (arrows).

He did not want to wear a total contact cast but agreed to continue to wear an Aircast. Repeat MRI after 3 months (Figure 3.3b) showed that there had been a reduction in the amount of marrow oedema and enhancement, particularly in the navicular, cuneiforms and second and third metatarsal bases. There remained some oedema through the cuboid. The Lisfranc ligament was identified and was slightly irregular. The foot gradually settled, casting was discontinued and he had no malalignment.

Learning points

- MRI can demonstrate bone marrow oedema and trabecular microfractures as early signs of Charcot foot.

- Total contact casting is the ideal treatment for the Charcot foot but a removable cast is also acceptable.

Case 3.4 Stress fractures

Charcot joints are often painless, but this patient first presented complaining of pain in the foot as well as redness and swelling following an injury to the toe.

This man was was 56 years old and had Type 1 diabetes for 17 years. He injured his left second toe and the injury was followed by redness, pain and swelling in his left foot. When he came to the Diabetic Foot Clinic as an emergency, the dorsal foot temperature was 3.2 °C greater than the same site on the contralateral foot. The skin was unbroken. X-ray was normal. A technetium diphosphonate bone scan showed increased activity in the left mid-foot in the region of the medial cuneiform, the first tarsometatarsal joint, and the left third metatarsophalangeal joint region (Figure 3.4a). He then had an MRI, which showed oedema and enhancement within the subchondral bone at the first tarsometatarsal joint and a stress fracture at the base of the first metatarsal (Figure 3.4b–d). He was treated in a total contact cast. He was notable for experiencing considerable pain and was treated with paracetamol and codeine. (We avoid using non-steroidal anti-inflammatories because of

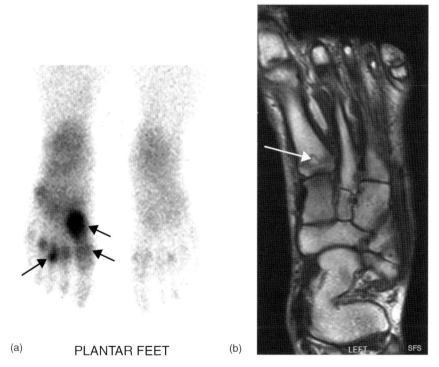

(a)   PLANTAR FEET   (b)

Figure 3.4 (a) Bone scan shows increased activity in the left mid-foot. In the region of the medial cuneiform, first tarsometatarsal joint and third metatarsophalangeal joint (arrows). (b) MRI T1 sequence showing a stress fracture at the base of the first metatarsal (arrow).

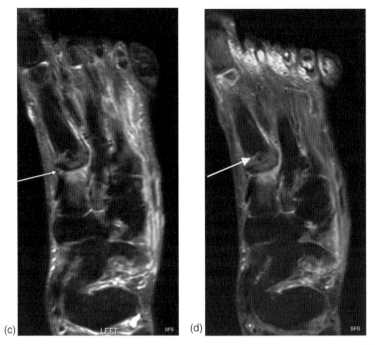

Figure 3.4 (*continued*) (c) MRI STIR sequence showing oedema and enhancement within the sub-chondral bone at the first tarsometatarsal joint (arrow). (d) MRI post-gadolinium sequence showing a stress fracture at the base of the first metatarsal (arrow).

the possible side-effects, including nephropathy.) By 6 months, his foot temperatures were within 2 °C of each other. On X-ray there was some remaining sclerosis and lucency of the tarsal bones.

Learning points

- The importance of early treatment in a cast should be emphasized. If the diagnosis cannot be confirmed by X-ray, then the patient should go into a removable cast until other investigations can be performed.

- Often the site of bone marrow oedema in the early Charcot foot is the subchondral region.

- Charcot feet although neuropathic may be painful.

Case 3.5   Casting for Charcot

As we have seen, diagnosing a Charcot joint early is not enough: if the patient fails to follow advice then destruction and deformity can be the outcome, as illustrated again in this case. We have seen patients who refuse to wear casts, or develop "cast phobia" and insist that they are removed. It is unfortunate when patients like this man develop an unrelated problem and blame it on the cast.

This 57 year old patient with Type 2 diabetes diagnosed for 4 years and painful neuropathy treated with gabapentin presented to the Clinic with a red swollen right foot, which was 4.4 °C warmer than his left foot. He had intact feet. A Duplex scan of his right lower leg ruled out a deep vein thrombosis. X-ray of his right foot revealed soft tissue swelling and evidence of an old fracture (Figure 3.5a) within the proximal phalanx of the right fifth toe with no further bony abnormality. The foot was at Stage 2. A blood test at presentation was carried out and CRP was 17.2 mg/l, WBC was 7.2×10^9/l, and glycated haemoglobin was 8%. Although X-ray at presentation was not indicative of early bone damage, a technetium bone scan revealed an increased uptake of isotope in the first and second tarsometatarsal joints, confirming the clinical diagnosis of Charcot foot (Figure 3.5b). The patient was treated with a total contact cast. He attended after one week for a routine cast check and all seemed well. However, three days later, the patient came back to the Clinic and asked for the cast to be removed as it was restricting his ability to wash prior to praying. His foot was still hot and swollen with a temperature difference of

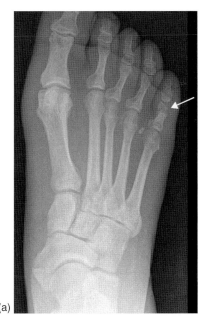
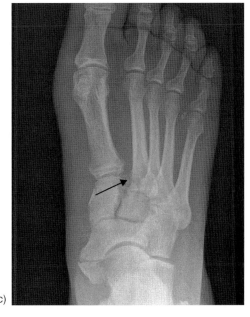

(a)   (c)

Figure 3.5   (a) X-ray with soft tissue swelling and old fracture of fifth toe (arrow). (c) X-ray shows LisFranc dislocation at the base of the second metatarsal (arrow).

Bone scan

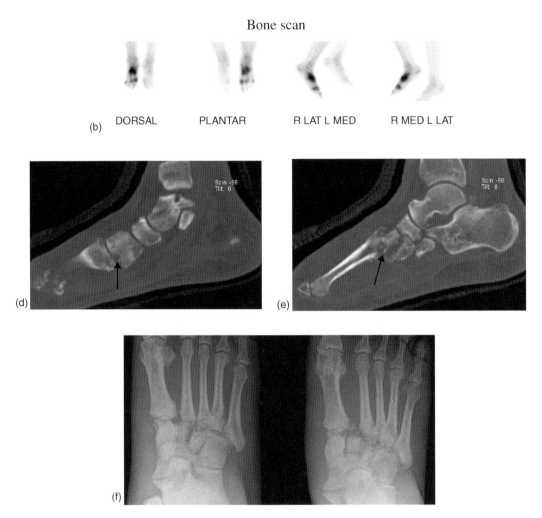

(b)

DORSAL   PLANTAR   R LAT L MED   R MED L LAT

(d)

(e)

(f)

Figure 3.5 (*continued*) (b) Bone scan shows increased uptake in the mid-foot and in the heads of the second and third metatarsal heads. (d) CT scan shows lucency and cystic changes associated with erosions in the first tarsometatarsal joint (arrow). (e) CT scan shows fracture of the second tarsometatarsal joint with multiple intra-articular bone fragmentation (arrow). (f) Final X-ray (straight and oblique) reveals extensive disorganisation of the tarsometatarsal joints.

4.2 °C between the feet. He was issued with a removable Aircast. A further X-ray was carried out at 3 weeks and this showed some lucency and disorganisation of the base of the second metatarsal, but apart from this the alignment of the mid-foot was maintained (Figure 3.5c). The patient was encouraged to continue casting treatment and he agreed to go back to total contact casting.

A CT of the mid-foot was arranged at this stage to reveal the extent of damage in the mid-foot. It showed lucency and cystic changes associated with erosions in the first tarsometatarsal joint, and a fracture of the second tarsometatarsal joint with multiple intra-articular bone fragmentation at the first and second tarsometatarsal joints (Figure 3.5d, e). A follow up X-ray at 6 weeks did not show any new damage compared with the X-ray at 4 weeks.

At 8 weeks, the patient returned as an emergency to the Diabetic Foot Clinic, complaining of pain in his right thigh, which he described as deep, gnawing and continuous day and night, and he blamed the cast. There was no allodynia or hyperpathia. Differential diagnosis included femoral neuropathy, but he was already taking gabapentin for painful neuropathy of the feet and lower legs. The pain of the right thigh, which was particularly worse at night, was so acute that he needed analgesia with morphine. Both knee jerks were absent. There was tenderness over the right quadriceps muscles. The CRP was normal. The problem was very localised over the mid quadriceps, and tender on palpation. Myonecrosis was suspected, the cast was removed and offloading with Aircast was offered. Creatine kinase was raised at 350 iu/l rising to 576 iu/l and then fell to 191 iu/l (normal is up to 150). The patient underwent MRI examination of the right thigh, which was normal, thus ruling out myonecrosis. MRI of the lumbar spine was also normal. The patient then had EMG examination, which showed evidence of a right femoral neuropathy.

At 12 weeks, his right foot was still 4.4 °C warmer compared with the contralateral foot. However, his X-ray did not reveal new damage and the patient was advised to continue the treatment with the Aircast. He then failed to attend for appointments at the clinic and was lost to follow-up until he came back to the clinic three months later. He admitted that he had discontinued wearing the Aircast and was wearing shoes. His right foot was swollen and 2.6 °C warmer than the left foot and had developed rocker bottom deformity. X-ray at this stage revealed extensive changes in the mid-foot with sclerosis, erosion and disruption of the distal tarsus associated with diastasis of the tarsometatarsal joints (Figure 3.5f).

Learning points

- This case reveals that early discontinuation of offloading for Charcot osteoarthropathy can lead to further bone and joint damage and development of subsequent foot deformity.

- The patient presented with acute Charcot osteoarthropathy and the diagnosis was made at the stage of a hot swollen foot with normal X-ray but abnormal bone scan.

- Treatment with casting over a period of 3 months held the alignment maintained, although it did not achieve complete healing of the fracture.

- His injudicious return to footwear and non-protected walking led to further extensive bone and joint destruction in the mid-foot with associated foot deformity.

- It is important to be persistent with casting treatment until there is clinical and radiological evidence of resolution. Patients require support and encouragement with this treatment.

- In the context of this case, the differential diagnosis of pain in the thigh was myonecrosis or femoral neuropathy. A normal MRI ruled out myonecrosis whereas EMG confirmed femoral neuropathy.

3.3   Different presentations

We now move to the different presentations seen in Charcot patients. We have recently noticed that Type 1 patients are more likely to present with fractures and Type 2 patients with dislocations. Another presentation in Type 1 patients is avascular necrosis.

3.3.1   Type 1 patients with osteopaenia

Case 3.6   A case of avascular necrosis involving the metatarsal heads

A 21 year old lady who had Type 1 diabetes of 15 years duration was being treated for anorexia nervosa. She was noted to have dorsal puffiness and swelling, involving first the left foot and then both feet. There was no associated discomfort and all pedal pulses were palpable. They were Stage 2 feet. X-ray showed deformity of the metatarsal heads with appearances suggestive of avascular necrosis, namely fragmentation and lucency of the second and third metatarsal heads of both feet (Figure 3.6). She was supplied with a wheelchair and her stay in the hospital enabled her to comply with a strict non-weight-bearing regime for 4 weeks. The oedema gradually resolved. Deformity did not develop and the radiological changes stabilized. The orthotist then made her bespoke shoes.

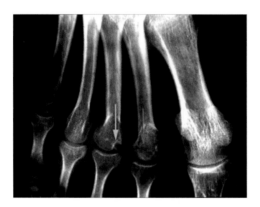

Figure 3.6   X-ray shows signs of avascular necrosis of metatarsal heads (arrows).

Learning point

- Charcot osteoarthropathy affecting the forefoot is characterised by radiological changes suggestive of avascular necrosis.

- Anorexia nervosa is a risk factor for both osteopaenia and avascular necrosis.

- Charcot foot may present spontaneously with no history of trauma.

Case 3.7   Multiple fractures and Charcot forefoot

Some unfortunate patients with thin bones develop multiple episodes of Charcot's osteoarthropathy affecting different sites.

This lady was 40 years old. She was a Type 1 diabetic patient diagnosed at the age of seven. She had amenorrhoea since the age of 16, and was underweight. She had severe generalised osteoporosis. On the left ankle she had had internal fixation of a fracture through the lower fibula. She had developed diabetic nephropathy and was started on CAPD and then underwent kidney–pancreas transplant. She was treated with corticosteroids for the first year post transplantation.

One year later, bone densitometry indicated that at the lumbar spine L2–L4 the bone mineral density (BMD) was 1.072 ± 0.01 g/cm^2, and the T score was -1.07 and the Z score was -0.64. BMD at the left femoral neck was 0.721 ± 0.01 g/cm^2 and the T score was -2.1; the Z score was -1.7. The T scores of the hip and spine were low and in the category for low bone mass. The hip readings were worse than the spine, with moderately increased risk of fracture. Three years later, her bone densitometry was repeated, which indicated that at the lumbar spine L2–L4 the BMD was 1.146 ± 0.01 g/cm^2, the T score was -0.6 and the Z score was -0.2. The left femoral neck showed that the BMD was 0.753 ± 0.01 g/cm^2 and the T score was -1.89; the Z score was -1.48. There was a 6.9 and 4.4% BMD increase in lumbar spine and left femur respectively over 3 years.

In the same year, she developed a painful right foot. She underwent X-ray locally and bone scan, both of which were reported as normal. However, when the pain failed to resolve two months later she was referred to the Diabetic Foot Clinic. The temperature of the foot was not raised. She had an X-ray, which showed loss of height of the right second and third metatarsal heads (Figure 3.7a). There was extensive sclerosis affecting the right tarsus. She was treated with an Aircast. The swelling settled after treatment in the Aircast.

BMD was repeated 3 years later and there was an 8% increase in lumbar spine BMD but a 3% decrease in mean total femur BMD. She was seen again 1 year later following an accident when she was knocked over, and was seen at a local hospital with an injury to her right ankle, but not X-rayed. We X-rayed her and there was an irregularity of the os calcis with surrounding sclerosis in keeping with a stress fracture (Figure 3.7b). She was treated again in an Aircast, but non-weight-bearing, and had a CT scan, which confirmed a fracture (Figure 3.7c). Later that year she had a fracture of the neck of the right femur, which was pinned locally. Her feet were at Stage 2 throughout these episodes.

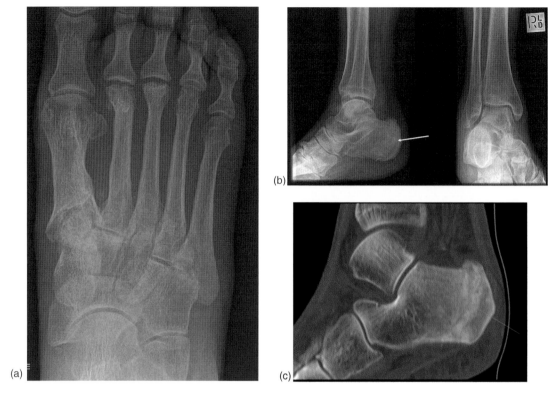

Figure 3.7 (a) X-ray shows loss of height of the second and third metatarsal heads and sclerosis of right tarsus. (b) Irregularity of the os calcis with surrounding sclerosis in keeping with a stress fracture (arrow). (c) CT scan indicates fracture of calcaneum (arrow).

Learning points

- This was a long standing Type 1 patient with osteopaenia of the lower limb.

- There was a gradual decrease in the BMD of the left femur. This predisposed her to pathological fracture.

- There should be a high index of suspicion of fracture and the possibility of an ensuing Charcot foot in all Type 1 diabetic patients, especially after minor trauma.

- Fractures in Type 1 diabetic patients need long immobilisation and casting because of slow healing of fractures in these patients.

Case 3.8 Osteopaenia and the neuropathic limb

This lady has been coming to the Diabetic Foot Clinic for many years, since her mother first brought her to us at the age of 16. She has multiple complications, and described her bones as being "like egg shells".

This 32 year old lady with Type 1 diabetes for 25 years first presented with a right swollen foot. A bone scan showed increased activity in the right hind foot and she was treated in a cast, and the foot settled in three months. She was then admitted one year later with ketoacidosis and infection of the chest wall and needed surgical drainage of a large abscess. Two years later she had a fracture of the lateral compartment of the left knee, leading to a Charcot knee. She had severe autonomic neuropathy in addition to her sensory neuropathy, and gastric emptying studies one year later after a labelled meal containing mashed potato and Dowex indicated that there was evidence of moderately severe gastroparesis.

In the same year, she developed a swollen right foot and X-ray showed erosive changes at the first, second and third metatarsophalangeal joints and a forefoot Charcot was diagnosed. She was casted and the swelling resolved after six months.

Two years later, she underwent bone densitometry. BMD at lumbar spine L2–L4 was 1.100 ± 0.01 gm/cm^2, T score $= -0.83$, Z score $= -1.00$. At the left femoral neck BMD was 0.811 ± 0.01 gm/cm^2, T score $= -1.40$, Z score -1.48. The hip T score was low and was in the category for low bone mass. The spinal readings were within normal range. Three years later, repeat bone densitometry showed a 0.5% loss of BMD in the spine and a 3.1% loss at the femur over the last three years. This was a normal spine result but femoral osteopaenia. The same year she complained of pain and swelling of the left heel. MRI showed a stress fracture at the posterior process of the left calcaneum (Figure 3.8a). Shortly after this, she developed a fracture of the right calcaneum (Figure 3.8b), and was treated in bilateral casts. A follow-up

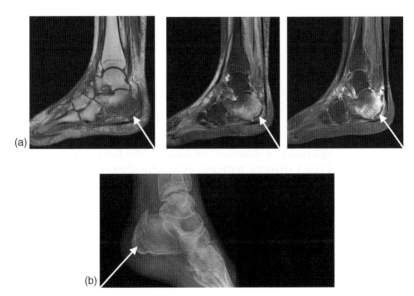

Figure 3.8 (a) MRI with T1 (left), STIR (middle) and post-gadolinium (right) sequences shows fracture of left calcaneum (arrows). (b) X-ray shows fracture of right calcaneum (arrow).

MRI one year later showed that the fracture through the posterior process of the left calcaneum could be identified but was almost healed, as was the contralateral fracture.

Learning points

- This was another Type 1 patient with osteopaenia of the lower limb.
- This led to susceptibility to fractures, including bilateral calcaneal fractures.
- She was not aware of traumatising either heel.
- Be aware of fracture in Type 1.
- Type 1 patients with osteopaenia and autonomic neuropathy are also susceptible to Charcot knee.

3.3.2 Infections in the Charcot foot

Case 3.9 "Foot 'flu"

A 38 year old man with poorly controlled Type 1 diabetes of 20 years' duration attended the Diabetic Foot Clinic. He had neuropathy with a VPT of more than 40 V. He fractured his right fifth metatarsal (Figure 3.9a). He was casted at his local hospital for 6 weeks. One year later, he complained of swelling in the right foot. X-ray revealed the old fracture of the base of the right fifth metatarsal bone with features of avascular necrosis affecting the navicular bone and the medial and intermediate cuneiforms and cuboid. He received a total contact cast (Figure 3.9b).

One year later, he visited his general practitioner complaining of malaise, tiredness, fever and poorly controlled diabetes. Influenza was common in the community at that time and the patient was advised to increase his insulin dose, take paracetamol and go to bed at home, and his wife was advised to test him for the presence of ketones. After 48 hours there was no improvement, the patient sweated very heavily and developed rigors, and when he got out of bed so that his wife could change the sheets she noticed redness and swelling of his right ankle and brought him immediately to the Diabetic Foot Clinic. His CRP was 100.0 mg/l but his WBC was normal at 6.99×10^9/l, neutrophils 4.80×10^9/l. He had a fever of 38.5 °C. There was no open lesion on the ankle, but he had an ulcer on the toe. On the ankle, fluctuant swelling was palpated (Figure 3.9c). This was a Stage 4 foot. He was seen by the orthopaedic surgeon, who aspirated thin watery pus from the area of fluctuance, which was sent for culture and subsequently grew a Group B haemolytic *Streptococcus* sensitive to ampicillin and penicillin (Figure 3.9d).

The patient categorically refused admission and was treated with IM ceftriaxone 1 g in 3.5 ml 1% lignocaine and bedrest at home. When the microbiology results were available a

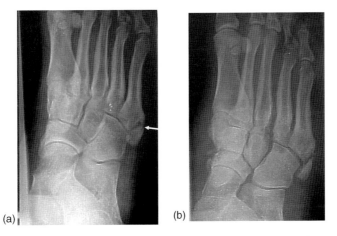

(a)   (b)

Figure 3.9 (a) X-ray shows fracture of base of fifth metatarsal (arrow). (b) X-ray shows the old fracture of the base of the right fifth metatarsal bone with features of avascular necrosis affecting the navicular bone and the medial and intermediate cuneiforms and cuboid.

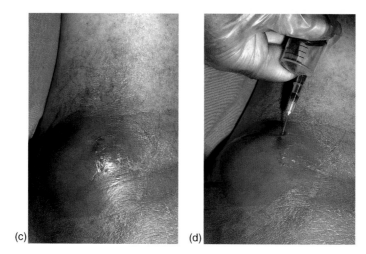

(c)   (d)

Figure 3.9 (*continued*) (c) Fluctuant swelling of the ankle. (d) Aspiration of ankle.

diagnosis of septic arthritis was made. He was urgently reviewed in the Foot Clinic. The swelling and redness had reduced and his temperature was normal. He continued to have IM ceftriaxone for one month. Further X-rays showed remaining sclerosis of the tarsal Charcot's osteoarthropathy, while the ankle remained normal.

   He was reluctant to attend the Foot Clinic regularly but his wife conducted a daily foot check looking for the presence of colour change, swelling, excessively hot or cold sites or painful areas. She brought him back to the Clinic four years later with a swollen left foot and he had a technetium diphosphonate bone scan, which showed increased uptake in the left mid-foot, and he received a total contact cast.

Learning points

- People with poorly controlled diabetes are prone to infection, and foot infections may present with symptoms of influenza. The feet and legs should always be inspected if the patient is unwell.

- Infection is unlikely if there is no break in the skin. However, some traumatic injuries are so small that the portal of entry cannot be clearly seen. Furthermore, the foot may heal over, sealing in micro-organisms, which multiply and lead to a severe infection.

- Aspiration and drainage of fluctuant swellings are essential.

- Pus associated with a streptococcal infection is frequently thin and watery in appearance.

Case 3.10   A nasty episode of sepsis in three sites

Sepsis will sometimes present concurrently in Charcot feet and other sites. A careful examination should be made to ensure that additional infections are not overlooked in the excitement of locating the first.

This lady was 50 years old with Type 2 diabetes of 14 years' duration. She had proliferative retinopathy, which underwent laser photocoagulation therapy. She was an obese lady referred from another hospital with a rocker bottom left Charcot foot and ulceration (Figure 3.10). This was a Stage 3 foot. She was total contact casted and needed several admissions for sepsis. The foot healed eventually in 12 months, after which she had several small recurrences of ulceration but no episodes of sepsis.

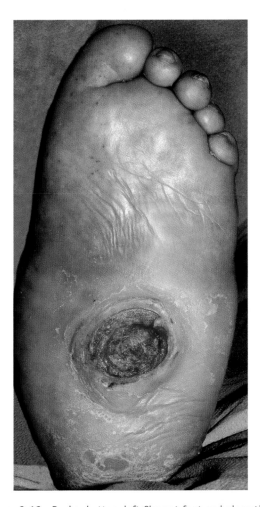

Figure 3.10   Rocker bottom left Charcot foot and ulceration.

Her foot ulcer recently recurred and she became unwell. She was admitted with lower abdominal pain, dysuria and frequency suggesting a urinary tract infection and a recurrence of the foot ulcer and infection. On presentation, her CRP was 235 mg/l, and her WBC was 17.45×10^9/l, of which 13.86×10^9/l were neutrophils. *Staphylococcus aureus* was grown from the foot and from both blood culture bottles. She also had multi-resistant *E. coli* and *Pseudomonas aeruginosa* in the foot, and the *E. coli* was also found in the urine. She was treated with vancomycin for staphylococcal septicaemia and foot infection (she was allergic to penicillin) and she was also treated with meropenem, to which the *Pseudomonas* and *E. coli* were sensitive. Although she had a staphylococcal bacteraemia she showed few signs of sepsis, having no fever. Infections in the blood, urine and foot all resolved on antibiotic therapy.

She had a further admission one month later with another urinary tract infection and was nauseated and vomiting. Urine showed heavy mixed growth and her foot ulcer grew *E coli*. She was treated with meropenem with resolution of her symptoms and was discharged after a few days.

Learning points

- This began as a life threatening episode of sepsis with *Staphylococcus aureus* cultured from the blood and from the foot. She also had a urinary tract infection with *E coli*. Eventually she had three sites of infection: the foot, the urine and the blood.

- Although she had a high white blood count she had no fever.

- She did not show the classical signs of sepsis, possibly because of her neuropathy.

3.3.3   Gout and the Charcot foot

The Charcot foot, infection and gout all present with redness, heat, swelling and sometimes pain. This can lead to considerable diagnostic problems.

Case 3.11   Gout or Charcot

This 68 year old man with Type 2 diabetes for 10 years and hypertension had been seen previously with "uncomfortable numbness", weakness and swelling in his feet. The VPT was 25 V on the right and 28 V on the left. EMG studies indicated that the right tibial nerve was inexcitable and the left tibial mean action potential was reduced in amplitude. The sural action potential was absent on both sides. There was a generalised sensory–motor neuropathy. He was treated with topical Opsite and responded well.

He then developed a left red, hot, swollen foot with palpable pulses (Figure 3.11a). He had a normal creatinine of 84 μmol/l and an eGFR of 83 ml/min. CRP was 34.5 mg/l.

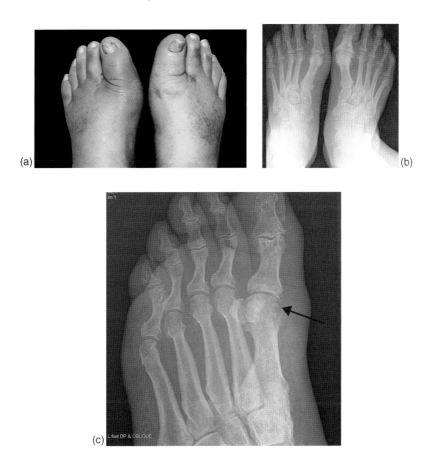

Figure 3.11   (a) Swollen red left foot. (b) X-ray of both feet reveals osteophyte formation, loss of joint space and subchondral cysts on the right first metatarsophalangeal joint and proximal interphalangeal joints. (c) X-ray of left foot shows erosions of first metatarsal head (arrow).

Uric acid was raised at 0.51 mmol/l. His WBC was 21.27×10^9/l with neutrophils of 16.56×10^9/l. On X-ray, the right first metatarsophalangeal joint and proximal interphalangeal joints were characterised by osteophyte formation, loss of joint space and subchondral cysts. There were also erosions of the first metatarsal head of the left foot (Figure 3.11b). The appearances indicated inflammatory arthropathy characterised by erosions suggestive of gout. This was a Stage 2 foot. He was treated with colchicine 500 µg bd and responded well.

Learning points

- The WBC can be greatly raised during acute episodes of gout.

- Serum uric acid is usually raised in gout but not always so.

- Bony erosions are a feature of gout but also Charcot foot.

Case 3.12   Gout or Charcot

This case described caused considerable difference of opinion among the Diabetic Foot Clinic team.

This lady was 53 years old with Type 2 diabetes of 12 years' duration. She had previously had thoracic spinal surgery for osteoporotic collapse. She developed, very suddenly, swelling, redness and pain around the first metatarsophalangeal joint spreading to the forefoot and involving the lower leg. She had undertaken a particularly intense period of housework and spring cleaning. She was already on long term diclofenac for her back, which had little effect. She also had a trial of colchicine, also with little effect. Subsequent serum uric acid was normal. The GP gave her several courses of antibiotics with no effect.

In the Diabetic Foot Clinic, she had an X-ray, technetium diphosphonate bone scan and CT scan. X-ray showed no evidence of erosions in the metatarsal head. She had a repeat X-ray 2 weeks later, which again showed no bony abnormality (Figure 3.12a). The bone scan showed markedly increased uptake in the first metatarsal head with some uptake in the shaft and base of the metatarsal. She then had a CT scan, which showed a large erosion in the first metatarsal head (Figure 3.12b). Her foot continued to be swollen and painful. Serum uric acid was 0.21 mmol/l on two occasions. She was treated as a Charcot foot and her foot put her in a total contact cast The swelling of the foot resolved. The foot remained at Stage 2 throughout.

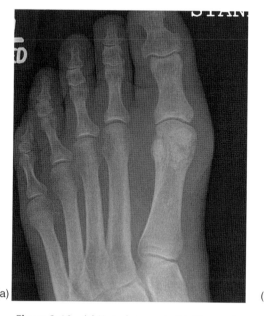

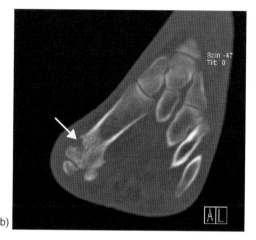

(a)   (b)

Figure 3.12   (a) X-ray is normal. (b) CT scan shows a large erosion in the first metatarsal head (arrow).

Learning points

- The diagnosis in this case was difficult: the differential was Charcot foot or gout.

- Charcot foot was favoured because the increased uptake on the bone scan involved not only the first metatarsophalangeal joint, but also the shaft and base.

- CT scan was useful in elucidating detail of bony damage and a large erosion of first metatarsal head.

- In this case CT revealed bony destruction not seen on X-ray.

Case 3.13 Swollen, painful knee: a problem of differential diagnosis

It should never be forgotten that two, or even three different conditions can exist in the same patient contemporaneously, each of which could account for the symptoms. The following patient had a red, hot, swollen foot, with a clearly infected burn on the dorsum, but there was more going on than infection, as will be seen: this was triple pathology involving three different sites in one leg.

An 70 year old Afro-Caribbean man with insulin treated Type 2 diabetes for 13 years, who had previously been seen at the Diabetic Foot Clinic with painful neuropathy, suffered a fall at home and developed swelling of his left foot. Following development of swelling he had discomfort in his foot and soaked it in hot water and developed a burn over the dorsum of the foot.

He then came to the Diabetic Foot Clinic as an emergency. This was a Stage 4 foot. He was admitted and treated with IV quadruple antibiotic therapy, amoxicillin 500 mg tds, flucloxacillin 500 mg qds, metronidazole 500 mg tds and ceftazidime 1 g tds. On admission his serum uric acid was noted to be 0.54 mmol/l with a normal creatinine of 106 μmol/l. The X-ray showed osteopaenia of the bones and flattening of the navicular (Figure 3.13a) and the MRI (Figure 3.13b) showed fracture and dislocation of the navicular and marrow oedema and enhancement affecting all the tarsometatarsal joints, involving the cunei-forms, the navicular, and the cuboid.

A diagnosis was made of Charcot's osteoarthropathy, and the aim was to heal the infected burn quickly (Figure 3.13c) so that he could be treated in a total contact cast. He responded quickly to treatment with antibiotics, rest and elevation: the burn was not full thickness and quickly healed. While initially his CRP increased from 78.3 to 85.5 mg/l, two days later it fell to 48.6 mg/l. Careful examination then revealed a left swollen knee, which was warm to touch and painful. His knee was aspirated and the fluid was cloudy and demonstrated uric acid crystals, and gout was diagnosed. He was treated with colchicine 500 μg bd for a week and the knee settled. After the burn healed his antibiotics were stopped and a total contact cast was applied.

Learning points

- Thirty percent of Charcot patients report pain or discomfort.

- Differential diagnosis can be a problem. Gout and Charcot foot may be triggered by a trauma.

- Charcot knee was also a possibility, but this is a rare complication, which we have only seen in patients with pre-existing, long-standing Charcot's osteoarthropathy involving the foot.

- CRP can rise during the first 24 hours despite starting treatment, as it reflects the inflammatory processes over the previous 24 hours.

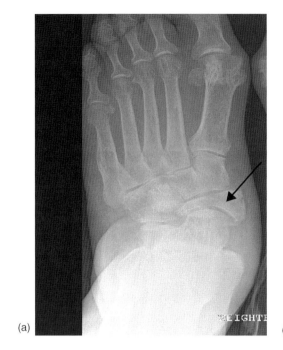

(a)

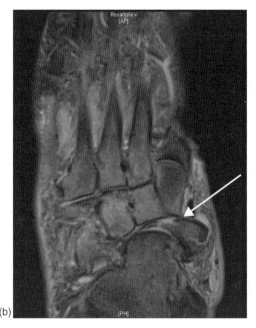

(b)

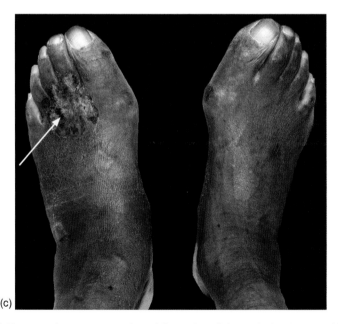

(c)

Figure 3.13 (a) The X-ray shows osteopaenia and flattening of the navicular (arrow). (b) MRI showing fracture and dislocation of the navicular (arrow) and marrow oedema and enhancement affecting all the tarsometatarsal joints, involving the cuneiforms, the navicular and the cuboid. (c) Healing burn of left foot (arrow).

3.3.4   *The neuroischaemic Charcot foot*

3.3.4.1   *Charcot foot that develops ischaemia*

Difficulties are encountered when a chronic, deformed Charcot foot develops ischaemia. We describe a patient who had been coming to the Diabetic Foot Clinic for many years, and although he could not be kept free of ulceration the situation was under control until ischaemia supervened.

Case 3.14   Neuropathy, ischaemia and the Charcot foot

A 63 year old man with Type 2 diabetes of 19 years' duration had severe co-morbidities, including retinopathy, chronic obstructive airways disease and psoriasis, and was morbidly obese. He was divorced and lived with his sons. He had Meniere's disease, with episodes of severe vertigo. He first became known to the Diabetic Foot Clinic team when he had neuropathic feet with bounding pulses and was referred to the Diabetic Foot Clinic by his general practitioner with bilateral Charcot feet with rocker bottom deformities. The feet were at Stage 2. He had a history of atrial fibrillation and an X-ray in 2000 showed an enlarged heart and bilateral perihilar oedema in keeping with cardiac failure. He had a long history of alcohol dependency. Liver ultrasound showed an enlarged liver and spleen. He had had several episodes of pneumonia. He saw the orthotists and was issued with bespoke boots with cradled insoles. X-rays of both feet showed disorganisation of the tarsal bones, which was more evident on the left than the right.

He did well until the foot pulses had become impalpable and he developed an ulcer over the fifth metatarsal head of the left foot (Stage 3 foot), which did not heal despite regular debridement in the Diabetic Foot Clinic and oral antibiotics. He was admitted to hospital and underwent an angioplasty of stenoses in the anterior and posterior tibial arteries, and these were dilated with a 4 mm balloon. There was also a stenosis in the peroneal artery, but the patient had severe pain in his back and said that he could no longer stay still, so the peroneal stenosis was not ballooned.

One year later, he developed an ulcer on his right heel and was admitted rather late with cellulitis (Stage 4 foot). Wound swabs grew MRSA and he was treated with IV vancomycin 1 g statim and then dosage according to serum levels. He was unable to wear a cast, but was given boots by the orthotist. He was unable to don and doff these without help, so there were many occasions when he walked around the house without shoes. He was not suitable for total contact casting in view of his propensity to develop severe sepsis, his obesity and his unsteadiness.

Later in that year, there was another admission with MRSA foot infection, again treated with vancomycin. We have always felt that in patients with indolent ulceration and recurring sepsis it is essential to optimise blood flow, so he again underwent angiography of both legs. On the right, anterior and posterior tibial vessels were of good calibre, and the peroneal was slightly attenuated. On the left there was a normal posterior tibial and normal anterior tibial. No angioplasty was done. The ulcer on his right heel persisted and he developed osteomyelitis on the background of a disorganised Charcot. Right foot X-ray showed destruction of the calcaneum with multiple bony fragments. There was sclerosis and loss of configuration within the subtalar and mid tarsal joints. The right heel ulcer eventually became very deep with bone exposed.

Persistent bleeding post-debridement was a problem in the Diabetic Foot Clinic. He was admitted to hospital. A swab grew *Klebsiella*, *Enterobacter* and MRSA and he was treated with IV vancomycin 1 g statim and then dosage according to serum levels and IV meropenem 1 g tds, which was then changed to tobramycin. He underwent surgical debridement and patial calcanectomy and was then seen by the plastic surgeon, who was happy to apply a skin graft, but the patient decided against this. He was eventually discharged on oral ciprofloxacin 500 mg bd and metronidazole 400 mg bd. He then stopped attending the Diabetic Foot Clinic but allowed the district nurses to visit him once a week.

His final admission was for an infected heel ulcer. He had vomited and became unwell at home. He had an endoscopy, and died suddenly the next morning on the ward. He had a post mortem, which showed congestive cardiac failure and cirrhosis of the liver.

Learning points

- This man developed Charcot's osteoarthropathy with deformity when he was a pure neuropath. Later, when he had developed multiple comorbidities, including ischaemia, it proved impossible to prevent and heal his ulcer.

- Every step should be taken to prevent and heal ulcers of the Charcot foot. Developing an ulcer on a Charcot foot is a pivotal event. Ulcers frequently prove very hard to heal and an ulcer on the hind foot can lead to disaster, as in this case.

- Bleeding can be a particular problem when debriding heel ulcers.

- There is a considerable mortality among Charcot patients.

3.3.4.2 Acute Charcot joint in a neuroischaemic foot

We have covered the problems that arise when ischaemia develops in a chronic Charcot foot, and now describe two extremely interesting and rare cases, where an acute Charcot joint has developed in an ischaemic foot. We have only seen these two cases in 29 years: all the other patients we have seen with acute Charcot feet had bounding pulses and well perfused feet, and we had believed that a well perfused foot was a prerequisite for the Charcot process. We still believe that, almost always, acute Charcot joints develop in a well perfused neuropathic foot with bounding pulses. However, we have seen these two cases of acute Charcot foot developing in patients with peripheral vascular disease, and they are described below.

Case 3.15   Acute Charcot foot in a neuroischaemic patient

This 70 year old man had Type 2 diabetes of ten years' duration, cryptogenic cirrhosis and an orthoptic liver transplant. His creatinine was 202 μmol/l. He took prednisolone 5 mg od and mycophenolate 750 mg bd. He also had sciatica and an MRI showed marked narrowing of the left neuro-exit foramen at L5/S1 due to osteophytes. He had an ulcer on the lateral aspect of the left lower leg. This was thought to be venous in origin. He had an erythema of venous congestion and was treated with compression stockings.

He presented with a hot swollen right leg and foot. This was a Stage 2 foot. X-ray showed a Lisfranc fracture dislocation (Figure 3.15a, b). He had impalpable pedal pulses, and underwent an arterial Duplex, which showed triphasic flow in iliac and femoral arteries and diffuse plaque in the popliteal artery with a tight stenosis in the anterior tibial artery at

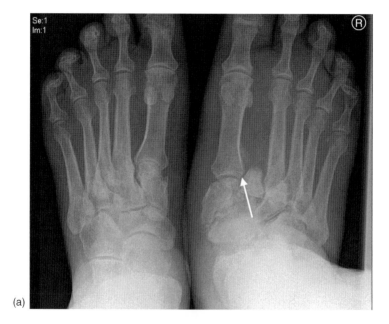

(a)

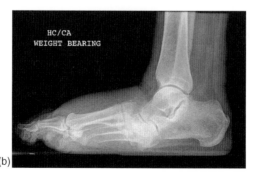

(b)

Figure 3.15   (a) X-ray of both feet, with Charcot foot on right with Lisfranc fracture-dislocation (arrow). (b) Lateral view of right foot reveals dislocation.

mid-calf with a fourfold increase in velocity, and there was moderate plaque in the tibioperoneal trunk and at the origin of the posterior tibial artery. He underwent tibial angioplasty and the foot was treated with a removable cast.

Learning points

- We believe that in this unusual case the administration of steroids post liver transplantation may have predisposed him to develop a Charcot foot.

- In this case, the peripheral vascular disease needed to be treated with angioplasty so that safe casting of the foot could be carried out.

Case 3.16   A long day's journey into night

A 62 year old man with Type 1 diabetes of 42 years' duration was referred to the Diabetic Foot Clinic five months after he suffered a myocardial infarction. He had attended annual review at the Diabetic Clinic, where the nurse had noticed a red patch with associated callus on the dorsum of his right second toe, together with a "nail problem" of the right first toe (Figure 3.16a). There was a hammer-toe deformity of the second toe and the prominent dorsum of the interphalangeal joint was subjected to pressure from an inadequate shoe with an overly narrow and shallow toe box. The problem of the first toenail was a Beau's line, a problem which is common in patients who undergo an episode of severe illness (in this case the myocardial infarction) when blood flow or nutrition of the nail bed is disrupted and growth of the nail is temporarily affected, resulting in the development of a deep transverse groove across the nail plate. Sometimes all the nails are affected, and sometimes only one nail, as in this case. This was a Stage 2 foot. The first nail was cut back, and a pair of bespoke shoes was provided. Two weeks later the second toe was greatly improved. His VPT was over 40 V, so he was offered regular foot care in the Diabetic Foot Clinic, which he accepted even though he lived 40 miles from the hospital.

Three months later a nail punctured the sole of his shoe and he sustained a trauma over the second metatarsal head. He attended the Foot Clinic the following day, and an area of blistering was debrided. This was a Stage 3 foot. The foot was cleaned and dressed and the foot healed in five days. The following year he developed callus over the same site, and an insole was manufactured and inserted into his shoe to offload the site. However, he came to the clinic with callus and signs of blistering (Figure 3.16b) and when the callus was debrided a small neuropathic ulcer was exposed. He refused a total contact cast but agreed to wear bespoke hospital shoes with cradled insoles, and the ulcer healed, but broke down again two months later after he had "walked a lot and run for a bus". The footwear was adjusted and the ulcer healed in three weeks.

He then did well for eight years, but his pedal pulses became weaker. He was asymptomatic and did not wish to be seen by the vascular team. The following year he attended the Foot Clinic for a routine appointment and it was immediately noted that he had developed severe deformity of the right foot with a prominence over the medial border of the foot where the overlying skin was blueish. He denied any trauma but said he had been on his feet a lot working as a guide. Charcot's osteoarthropathy was diagnosed: this was a very unusual case of Charcot in an ischaemic foot, which was confirmed by X-ray and bone scan. The orthopaedic surgeons were consulted as to the feasibility of taking him to theatre and attempting to reduce the medial dislocation and deformity, but they felt it would be unwise to attempt this. He developed severe rocker bottom deformity in addition to the existing medial convexity. He soon noticed a deep medial ulcer where the skin had been blue and plantar ulceration over the rocker-bottom deformity, despite treatment with a total contact cast.

His progress was stormy, necessitating several hospital admissions. He had a previous history of eczema and developed severe eczema under the stocking distribution area covered by the cast. The dermatologists felt that he might be sensitive to some of the casting

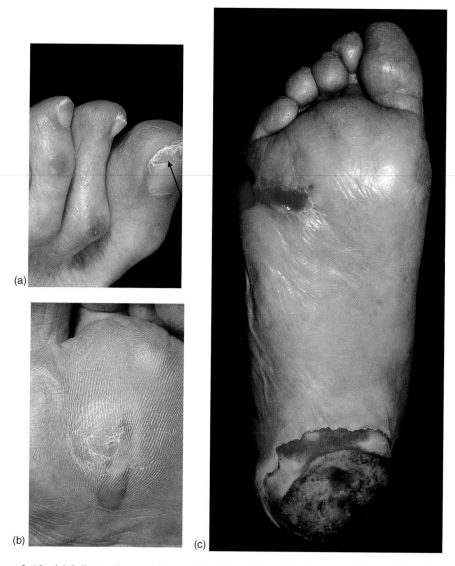

Figure 3.16   (a) Callus on dorsum of second toe. Beau's line of the first toe nail (arrow) (b) Callus with underlying ulcer. (c) Infected heel ulcer.

materials used, and before a cast was applied his leg was wrapped with zinc oxide bandage (Calorband) and was protected with three layers of stockinette under the casting materials, and the leg eczema healed and did not recur. A removable bivalved cast was made, followed by a Charcot Restraint Orthotic Walker, and the foot finally healed after two and a half years.

The main problem in his final year was right heel ulceration and impaired renal function aggravated by infection of the foot. He developed recurrent heel ulceration and he was admitted for tibial angioplasty. There were stenoses in the right peroneal artery, which was the only artery in the mid to distal calf. The stenoses were dilated with a 3 mm balloon. The anterior tibial artery was severely diseased, occluding in the upper calf. He had another admission for the right heel ulcer, which was infected with *Enterobacter cloacae*, *Pseudomonas aeruginosa* and *E. coli*. His creatinine was 527 µmol/l, having been 277 µmol/l one month previously. His CRP was 91.7 mg/l, but his WBC was only $8.01 \times 10^9/l$ and neutrophils $5.70 \times 10^9/l$. The creatinine fell to 148 µmol/l after IV meropenem 500 mg od and IV fluids and the CRP fell to 31.3 mg/l. He was readmitted after only six days at home, infected, and growing *Enterobacter cloacae* sensitive to meropenem, and mixed anaerobes (Figure 3.16c). His CRP was 94.3 mg/l with creatinine of 332 µmol/l, a white count of $9.00 \times 10^9/l$ and neutrophils of $5.57 \times 10^9/l$. He was treated again with IV meropenem, and his creatinine fell to 258 µmol/l and his CRP to 15.3 mg/l. He underwent another angiogram to ascertain whether there had been any deterioration in his vascular status, but no significant change was found.

In his final admission, he was readmitted with further sepsis, CRP of 119.3 mg/l, white blood count $6.6 \times 10^9/l$, neutrophils $3.73 \times 10^9/l$ and creatinine of 529 µmol/l. He had haemodialysis, but he suddenly deteriorated and went into pulmonary oedema and died.

Learning points

- Beau's lines are not dangerous, but any loose area of nail plate should be cut back and smoothed off to avoid it catching on the sock and traumatizing the toe.

- When patients are sensitive to casting materials the skin should be carefully protected from contact with them.

- Charcot's osteoarthropathy is very rare in the ischaemic foot but may occasionally be seen.

- In his final year, right heel ulceration in the Charcot foot and impaired renal function aggravated by infections of the foot were responsible for his demise.

3.4 Surgery

It is in the area of surgery that some of the most positive advances have been made in the management of the Charcot foot.

3.4.1 Internal fixation

Case 3.17 Operative internal stabilisation

This 53 year old man had Type 2 diabetes of 19 years' duration, and autonomic and peripheral neuropathy, and had strong pedal pulses and a VPT of over 50 V bilaterally when he first presented. He had proliferative bilateral diabetic retinopathy, treated by laser photocoagulation. He was referred to the Diabetic Foot Clinic with bilateral Charcot feet and bilateral plantar ulcers. These were Stage 3 feet. On the left foot there was a healed fracture of the left fifth metatarsal. Creatinine was 113 µmol/l, with eGFR 62 ml/min. He was very anxious, was reluctant to allow his feet to be debrided and refused plaster casts. He was an irregular attender, with long gaps in treatment, and he had recurrent ulceration.

He developed ulceration on the lateral aspect of the right mid-foot, having been previously admitted to his local hospital for IV antibiotics. X-ray showed a fracture of the base of the right fifth metatarsal (Figure 3.17a). He had an excision of an osteomyelitic base of the fifth metatarsal of the right foot and debridement of the ulcer, following which he had a reactivation of the Charcot process in the right foot, and then developed tibiotalar and subtalar joint instability. This led to recurrent inversion injuries and he was seen at the Joint Orthopaedic/Diabetic Foot Clinic. There was severe lateral ligamentous laxity with a fixed varus deformity of the hind foot (Figure 3.17b). He was initially treated with bracing but developed a pressure ulcer over the lateral border of the mid-foot. There was some collapse of the medial arch and it was planned to perform an acute corrective fusion of the subtalar joint. Ideal treatment would be to hold the deformity corrected in a frame to heal the ulcer and then to perform a mid-foot osteotomy to keep the foot in position. An alternative would be a tibiotalar nail. We were concerned about his social circumstances and did not think that he would cope with surgery involving offloading as he lived alone. Nor did we think that he would manage in a Taylor Spatial Frame without damaging either the frame or the foot. His sister then agreed to come and live with him.

He therefore underwent corrective tibiocalcaneal fusion of the right ankle with an intramedullary nail in the distal right tibia and screws in the calcaneum (Figure 3.17c). He was initially non-weight-bearing for three months and then partially weight-bearing in a bivalved plaster, and the deformity was corrected (Figure 3.17d).

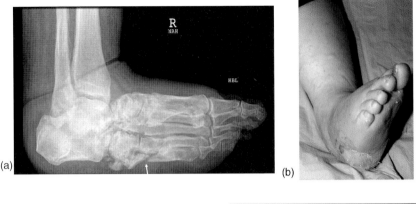

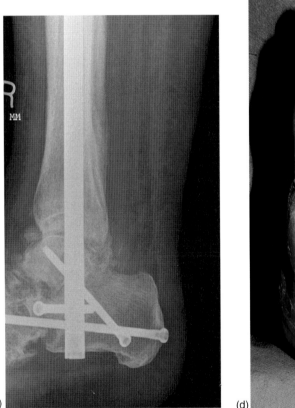

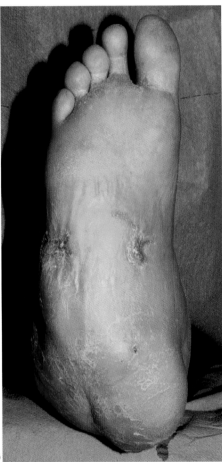

Figure 3.17 (a) X-ray shows fracture of base of right fifth metatarsal (arrow). (b) Varus deformity of the hind foot. (c) Postoperative X-ray intramedullary nail in the distal right tibia and screws in the calcaneum. (d) Good correction of varus deformity.

Learning points

- Previous osteomyelitis of the fifth metatarsal base and subsequent surgery had resulted in an inversion deformity of his existing Charcot foot.

- It was difficult to accommodate this long term with orthoses.

- Acute surgical correction was a successful alternative.

Case 3.18   A screw loose...

This was a lady who underwent internal stabilisation, and was the recipient of a kidney–pancreas transplant. She was referred very late to the Diabetic Foot Clinic for a second opinion after she had been told that amputation of her Charcot ankle was inevitable.

This 40 year old lady had Type 1 diabetes and received a kidney–pancreas transplant. She was seen in the Diabetic Foot Clinic and was very upset, tearful and anxious. She had had a bimalleolar fracture to the left ankle. Surgery was delayed due to the presence of MRSA in a right foot ulcer, and she developed a severe inversion deformity of the left ankle. She was then advised to have a left below the knee amputation but refused and was desperate to keep her leg. She had a longstanding ulcer on the plantar surface of her right foot, which had recently become worse and she had been advised to have that leg amputated as well.

She then asked to come to King's. She had a severe varus deformity of the left ankle (Figure 3.18a) and on the right side she had prominent metatarsophalangeal joints on the plantar aspect and a non-healing ulcer over the second metatarsophalangeal joint. This was a Stage 3 foot. We first treated her with a total contact cast to heal the ulcerated right foot and she had a left tibiocalcaneal fusion (Figure 3.18b). She was non-weight-bearing for six weeks. Unfortunately, the screws that had been inserted in the foot became loose and moved. There was migration of the distal locking screw and the orthopaedic surgeons thought that it would be necessary to adjust it surgically. However, on review one month later, no further migration of the screw had occurred, and the fixation was regarded as optimal, so further surgery was not needed. She remains ulcer free with a plantigrade foot (Figure 3.18c).

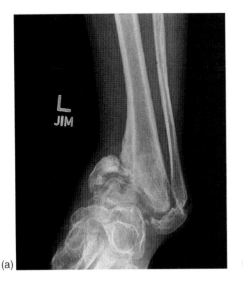

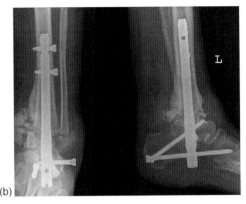

Figure 3.18   (a) X-ray of varus deformity of left ankle with disorganisation of the hind foot. (b) X-ray of left tibiocalcaneal fusion with intramedullary nail and screws.

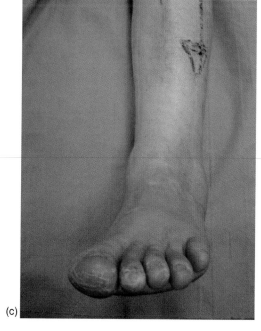

Figure 3.18 (*continued*) (c) Plantigrade foot.

Learning points

- Hind foot deformity can now be surgically corrected in the Charcot foot.

- Even though the patient may have considerable co-morbidity, such corrections can be successful if there is good coordination of multidisciplinary care, with particular attention paid to the postoperative wounds.

- Unstable hindfoot Charcot deformity is no longer an inevitable reason for major amputation.

3.4.2 External fixation

> ### Case 3.19 Stabilisation with frame followed by internal fixation

In addition to internal fixation, some patients benefit first from correction of their foot deformity and instability by using an external frame. Once corrected, relapse is prevented by internal fixation.

This 43 year old lady with Type 1 diabetes for 30 years was admitted with infected ulcers on her deformed right foot. This was a Stage 4 foot (Figure 3.19a). Wound swabs grew MRSA and she was started on IV vancomycin via a PICC line, and underwent debridement of the ulcers by the orthopaedic surgeons. She was discharged on teicoplanin 200 mg od. Four months later she was admitted for application of a Taylor Spatial Frame to the right foot for cavovarus Charcot deformity (Figure 3.19b) and two months later, she underwent a right mid-foot fusion with a bone graft from the right iliac crest and insertion of an intramedullary nail (Figure 3.19c, d). All was well at review, and she had a below knee bivalved cast.

However, she then developed a fracture in her calcaneum and needed right foot Charcot joint salvage surgery for failed fixation and fractured calcaneum (Figure 3.19e). She underwent right foot calcaneal and ankle fixation and demineralised bone matrix was introduced to the subtalar and ankle joint after denuding the ankle surfaces (Figure 3.19f), two screws were used to fix the ankle joint and a plate was applied to the calcaneum. The nail was left in for stability. Fixation was satisfactory. She was non-weight-bearing for three months. The hind-foot was holding well with no evidence of disruption of the calcaneum or the subtalar joint. She was allowed to weight-bear.

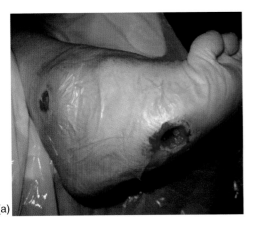

(a)

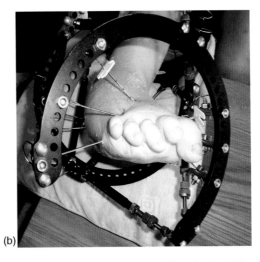

(b)

Figure 3.19 (a) The foot at presentation, with deformity and ulceration. (b) Foot with Taylor Spatial Frame.

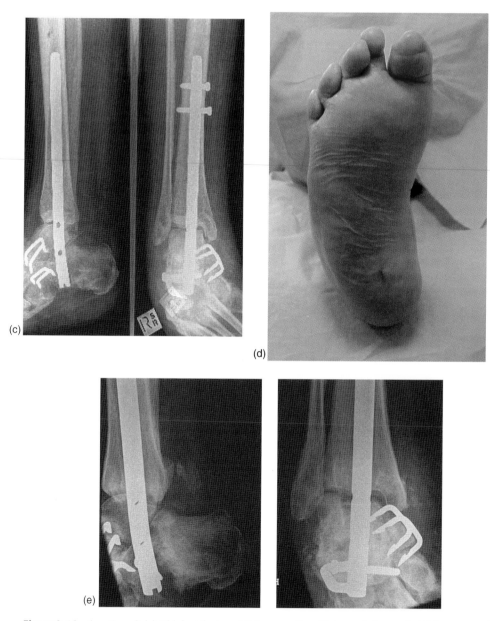

(c)

(d)

(e)

Figure 3.19 (*continued*) (c) Mid-foot fusion with bone graft and intramedullary nail. (d) Post correction the foot is plantigrade. (e) Failed fixation and fractured calcaneum.

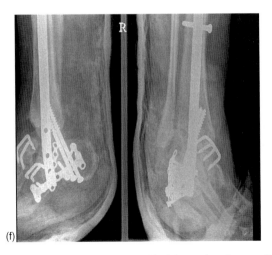

Figure 3.19 *(continued)* (f) Screws inserted to fix ankle joint and a plate applied to the calcaneum.

Learning points

- Reconstruction surgery is possible in diabetic patients with neuropathy but they are prone to several complications.

- Patients need considerable fortitude to undergo this lengthy and gruelling treatment; much moral support will be needed from the staff of the Diabetic Foot Clinic.

- Surgical procedures involve months of care, close supervision, and rapid action when problems develop.

Case 3.20 Hindfoot reconstruction avoiding amputation; care of postoperative wounds

The vulnerability to complications of Charcot patients undergoing surgery is extreme. We now describe the surgical course of a very frail lady.

This 60 year old lady had Type 2 diabetes of 18 years' duration. She fractured her ankle and developed a varus hind foot deformity. She had been aware of an injury but a fracture had not been diagnosed previously. She had a marked varus deformity of the hind foot of 45° with no major compensatory forefoot pronation. She had a chronic non-healing ulcer on the lateral aspect of the ankle joint (Figure 3.20a), and was wheelchair bound. She had a suprapubic catheter to treat her urinary incontinence.

On review of the history, the initial injury was a simple fall at home followed by progressive deformity leading to ulcerating lateral malleolus. She was considered for gradual corrective fusion of the ankle using a Taylor Spatial Frame, but she was not suitable for frame management, and said that she could not cope with a circular frame. Thus, she underwent acute corrective surgery. Post-operatively she had wounds on the plantar aspect of the heel, the apex of the heel (Figure 3.20b) and the lateral aspect of the lower leg and ankle (Figure 3.20c). Wound swabs grew *Pseudomonas aeruginosa* and she was treated with ciprofloxacin 500 mg bd orally and then IV piperacillin–tazobactam 4.5 g tds when a PICC line was inserted. Special removable casts to accommodate these wounds were made in the Diabetic Foot Clinic

Following insertion of the PICC line her CRP rose to 122 mg/l and three days later she developed fever, and had spiking temperature of 39.3 °C. The chest X-ray was normal. Piperacillin–tazobactam was stopped and she was treated with IV vancomycin 1 g statim and then dosage according to levels, IV gentamicin 320 mg statim and IV meropenem 1 g tds. She became confused, with low blood pressure of 90/50 mm Hg. Her suprapubic catheter was changed. The foot did not look infected and the wounds were healing well. The foot swab was negative. Further blood cultures taken from

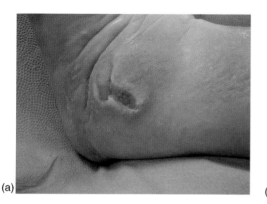

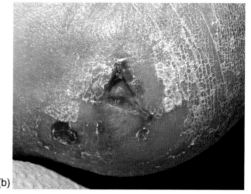

(a)   (b)

Figure 3.20 (a) Ulcer on ankle with varus deformity. (b) Wounds on the plantar aspect of the heel and the apex of the heel.

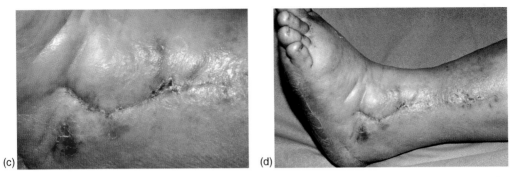

(c)   (d)

Figure 3.20 *(continued)* (c) Wound on lateral aspect of the lower leg and ankle. (d) Deformity is corrected and ulcer has healed.

the PICC line grew MRSA and she was given IV linezolid 600 mg bd and rapidly improved, with resolution of fever and reduction of CRP. A new PICC line was inserted. She was advised to be non-weight-bearing for at least 3–6 months. The foot healed (Figure 3.20d).

Learning points

- The patient had post-operative wound breakdown following acute corrective surgery.
- She needed a special removable cast to accommodate these wounds.
- The wounds also became infected and needed IV antibiotic therapy.
- These wounds put the success of the surgical correction at risk. They needed aggressive therapy.
- Diabetic patients are immunosuppressed and are susceptible to IV line infections.

Case 3.21 Charcot foot, Taylor Spatial Frame and pregnancy

This case, of a lady who also underwent external fixation, was the only case we have ever encountered of a patient with a Charcot foot and ulceration who became pregnant.

This lady was 34 years old and had Type 1 diabetes since the age of 13, and was a young mother, with a small child and a very hectic life. She had treated hypertension, and to control her diabetes she was on a subcutaneous insulin pump. She had proliferative retinopathy, which had laser photocoagulation nephropathy and chronic anaemia.

She had had a miscarriage. She then attended the Pre-Conception Counselling Clinic, where she was noted to have a Charcot left foot and ulceration and was referred to the Diabetic Foot Clinic for joint care between the Diabetic Department and the obstetricians. Her Charcot foot involved the tarsometatarsal joints, with sclerosis and marginal erosions and a dropped arch and severe rocker bottom deformity. She told us that she had had numerous ulcers and infections in the past, and the current ulcer had been present for several months. This was a Stage 3 foot. She was reluctant to take antibiotics, and said that she had multiple allergies, but she agreed to accept special shoes and these were made. Four months later, she was pregnant and became one of only four patients we have seen with foot ulceration in pregnancy. She had a baby boy and the foot remained ulcerated throughout the pregnancy despite intensive conservative management

In view of her long history of recurrent ulcerations and infections, and the severe foot deformity, she was seen by the orthopaedic surgeons and offered treatment to correct the deformity and stabilise the foot. She underwent external fixation with a Taylor Spatial Frame and osteotomy to the left foot. She had one episode of infection (Stage 4 foot) but this responded to IV antibiotics. Six months later, the frame was removed with the foot showing good consolidation and no further correction was needed. She was followed up in the Diabetic Foot Clinic.

Learning points

- Recurrent ulceration associated with deformity is an indication for surgery.

- Diabetic foot ulceration is rare in pregnancy.

- It should be managed with intensive conservative treatment with regular callus removal and specialised off-loading.

Case 3.22   Stabilisation with complications

This case developed complications with a Taylor Spatial Frame leading to sepsis. Although he was systemically unwell and needed admission, prompt treatment with IV antibiotics prevented further damage and it was not necessary to remove the frame and its pins.

The patient was 61 years old, and had Type 2 diabetes for 20 years. He developed a Charcot left foot with medial deformity. There was also an ankle varus deformity with a neuropathic ulcer. This was a Stage 3 foot. After passing through the active phase of his Charcot, the patient was considered for a Taylor Spatial Frame to correct the malalignment. Two weeks after applying this the ulcer had healed, but the patient developed nausea and anorexia and became unwell with a fever of 37.3 °C. CRP was raised at 120.3 mg/l, with serum creatinine of 145 μmol/l, with white count of 10.91×10^9/l and neutrophils 7.22×10^9/l. There was cellulitis on the dorsum of the foot with discharge from a pin site (Figure 3.22). A swab from the pin site grew *Pseudomonas aeruginosa* sensitive to ciprofloxacin and *Proteus vulgaris*, also sensitive to ciprofloxacin. There was no other obvious source of sepsis. The areas around the insertion of the pins were necrotic and an

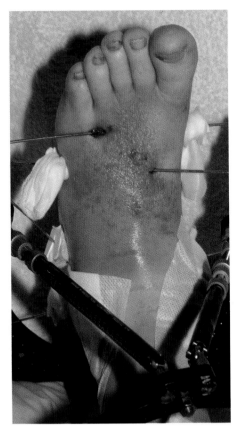

Figure 3.22   Cellulitis on the dorsum of the foot resulting from pin site infection.

infection was presumed. The patient was treated with IV meropenem 1 g tds. The fever settled and the nausea gradually improved and the CRP fell to 22.1 mg/l. The creatinine settled at 97 µmol/l. The pins were later removed at the appropriate time, according to the original plan, and he then underwent acute correction and insertion of a retrograde nail with a successful result.

Learning points

- Classical signs of infections are diminished in the diabetic patient and it is difficult to detect the signs of skin infections and particularly pin site infection.

- The CRP is a good indicator of inflammation and indirect indicator of the presence of infection.

- Although a pin site infection was diagnosed, this resolved with antibiotic therapy and there was no need to remove the pins.

- A diabetic patient with evidence of sepsis and a Taylor Spatial Frame should be closely examined for pin site infection.

- The results achieved with the Taylor Spatial Frame can be spectacular, but only if careful attention is paid to rapid detection and treatment of complications in the diabetic patient.

Case 3.23   Fixation and complications

This 60 year old patient had Type 2 diabetes. He had moderate renal impairment, with a creatinine of 150–160 µmol/l and multiple comorbidities. He had a past history of non-Hodgkin's lymphoma, which was in remission, ischaemic heart disease with a triple heart bypass in 1995, and spinal stenosis, which was operated on in 2002. He was referred to the Diabetic Foot Clinic with a Charcot foot with a rocker bottom deformity in 2004. This was a Stage 3 foot. He was concerned about the appearance of the foot and wished to have surgical correction of his rocker bottom deformity. He had an ulcer.

He was electively admitted for correction of the rocker bottom deformity. He had a mid-foot osteotomy and an application of a Taylor Spatial Frame. He had an episode of chest pain and shortness of breath post operatively, and had a raised D dimer, which did not rule out a pulmonary embolus. However, a CT pulmonary angiogram was negative, ruling out pulmonary embolus. The serum troponin was not raised, ruling out a myocardial infarction.

After discharge his creatinine rose to 260 µmol/l and two days later he was admitted to the orthopaedic ward with an infected diabetic foot ulcer. This was a Stage 4 foot. *Enterobacter aerogenes* was isolated from the foot, and he was treated with IV meropenem 500 mg bd and discharged five days later, when his serum creatinine had fallen to a normal level at 114 µmol/l. Ten days later he became unwell with shivering and pain in the heel. He was readmitted to the orthopaedic ward with ulcers secondary to the Taylor Spatial Frame, and fluid retention and disturbed renal function. Clinically he also developed cardiac failure. Echocardiogram showed raised right ventricular pressure of 35–40 mm Hg and a low normal left ventricular injection fraction. The serum creatinine was 259 µmol/l, potassium was 7.8 mmol/l, CRP was 45.0 mg/l and his WBC was normal at 8.21×10^9/l with neutrophils of 5.99×10^9/l.

His hyperkalaemia was treated with insulin and dextrose. A foot specimen grew *Morganella morganii* and *Stenotrophomonas maltophilia*. He responded to IV co-trimoxazole 460 mg bd. Within ten days, the creatinine had fallen to 120 µmol/l, the CRP had fallen to 7.9 mg/l and the frame was removed. He was followed up in the Diabetic Foot Clinic in a total contact cast, but complete healing was not achieved and the patient underwent exostectomy, after which he healed.

Learning points

- Diabetic patients in a Taylor Spatial Frame are susceptible to pin site infections, just as to infections elsewhere.

- Aggressive antibiotic treatment is needed.

- Pin site infections in the Charcot foot patient can destabilise the patient by aggravating renal and cardiac function.

- This patient had suffered life-threatening renal decompensation following infection. He needed IV insulin and glucose: with any potassium above 7 mmol/l there is a risk of irreversible arrhythmias.

3.4.3 *Exostectomy*

For many years the only elective surgery performed on Charcot patients at King's was exostectomy, to remove or shave bony prominences complicated by neuropathic ulceration. The beneficial results of this simple procedure are long term.

Case 3.24   Treatment of Charcot ulcer with exostectomy

A 62 year old man with Type 1 diabetes of 29 years' duration was referred to the Diabetic Foot Clinic from his local hospital, who had been treating his Charcot foot. Four years previously he had gone there in emergency with a red, hot, swollen foot. He was issued with crutches and advised to keep off the foot because there was a fracture, but because the foot was not painful he was told that a cast would not be necessary. Over the next months the foot changed shape, developing a rocker bottom deformity with a medial convexity, and he developed a large neuropathic ulcer (Figure 3.24a), which did not heal despite a two week long hospital admission for bedrest.

On examination his VPT was above 50 V bilaterally and his foot pulses were palpable. The ulcer on his foot appeared infected, with a thin discharge and musty odour, and a probe could be passed to underlying bone. This was a Stage 4 foot. He was admitted for IV antibiotics amoxicillin 500 mg tds, flucloxacillin 500 mg qds, metronidazole 500 mg tds and ceftazidime 1 g tds, and underwent surgical debridement and exostectomy of the underlying bony prominence. Bone cultures grew *Staphylococcus aureus* and he was treated with IV flucloxacillin 1 g qds and sodium fusidate 500 mg tds orally. He remained in hospital until full healing was achieved (Figure 3.24b).

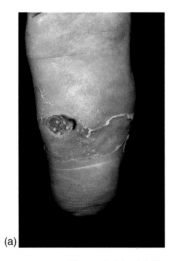
(a)

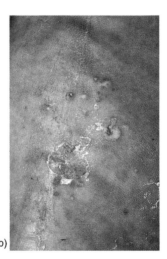
(b)

Figure 3.24   (a) Neuropathic ulcer. (b) The foot has healed.

Learning points

- It is a great mistake to refrain from casting fractures in the diabetic foot because the patient does not complain of pain.

- Many Type 1 patients with foot fractures are at the early stages of acute Charcot's osteoarthropathy.

- Bony prominences that become infected should be treated with exostectomy.

Case 3.25 They that endure to the end shall be saved

This case is of a man with very long-standing ulceration over a bony prominence on a severely deformed Charcot foot. His indolent six year old ulcer healed rapidly after exostectomy, where total contact casting had not been successful.

A 66 year old man with Type 2 diabetes for 12 years treated with insulin, hypertension, background retinopathy and a five year history of Charcot's osteoarthropathy was referred to the Diabetic Foot Clinic with an indolent plantar ulcer, which had been present for six years. He had a severe rocker bottom deformity. He was treated with a total contact cast but the ulcer was very slow to respond. He developed cellulitis of the foot and was admitted for IV antibiotics. He was treated with quadruple antibiotics given intravenously, amoxicillin 500 mg tds, flucloxacillin 500 mg qds, metronidazole 500 mg tds and ceftazidime 1 g tds. Swabs and tissue grew *Enterobacter* species sensitive to ciprofloxacin, which replaced the other antibiotics. It was a short admission because the patient was determined to go home as soon as possible.

Despite the long-term treatment in a cast, the ulcer failed to heal. He was reluctant to be admitted at King's again since he lived over 100 miles away, but finally agreed that he could not go on as he was. He was then seen in the Joint Orthopaedic/Diabetic Foot Clinic and put on the waiting list. He was admitted for exostectomy (Figure 3.25a, b). The

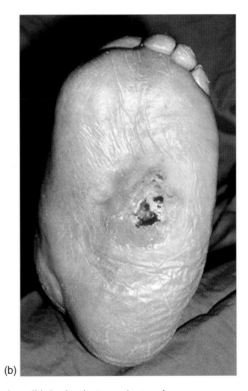

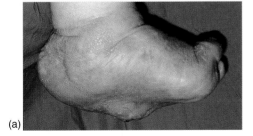

(a)

(b)

Figure 3.25   (a) Rocker bottom lateral view. (b) Rocker bottom plantar view.

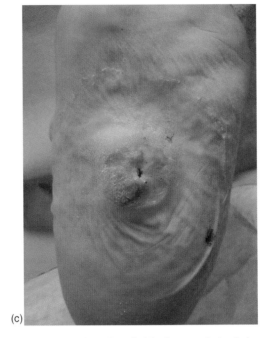
(c)

Figure 3.25 *(continued)* (c) Ulcer nearly healed.

rocker bottom foot was debrided and the entire navicular was removed. The bone specimen grew *Enterococcus faecium* and he was treated with IV teicoplanin 400 mg daily. He eventually healed (Figure 3.25c).

Learning points

- Rocker bottom plantar ulcers are very difficult to heal.
- It is reasonable to try total contact casting first as well as aggressive treatment of infection.
- They may need prolonged casting and often exostectomy.

Case 3.26   Infection, deformity and the Charcot Foot

This 61 year old man had Type 2 diabetes of 7 years' known duration. He was referred to the Diabetic Foot Clinic with bilateral midfoot Charcot feet. He was admitted for treatment of an infected ulcer on the medial convexity of his right foot. This was a Stage 4 foot. On admission his CRP was 167 mg/l, but his WBC was normal, at 8.77×10^9/l. He underwent surgical debridement. The bone specimen grew *Enterobacter cloacae* and *Enterococcus faecalis* and he was given IV amoxicillin 1 g tds and oral ciprofloxacin 500 mg bd. He was discharged with a CRP of 10 mg/l but was re-admitted two weeks later with a CRP of 142 mg/l, spreading cellulitis and osteomyelitis of the right foot (Figure 3.26a). He underwent a further debridement in theatre with removal of infected bone and shaving of the bony prominence. The bone specimen sent from theatre grew *Cornebacterium striatum* sensitive to amoxicillin. He healed quickly, has not relapsed (Figure 3.26b) and remains under the long term management of the Diabetic Foot Clinic.

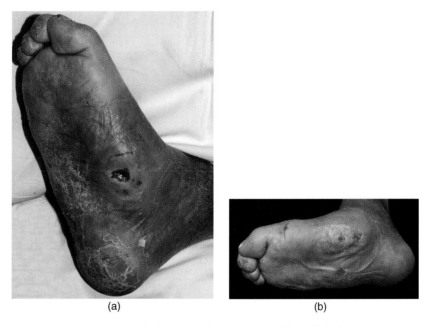

(a)   (b)

Figure 3.26   (a) Infected ulcer on medial convexity. (b) Healed after exostectomy.

Learning points

- Exostectomy can have the thrice useful role of removing infected bone and also bony prominence and providing bone specimens for culture and accurate antibiotic therapy.
- The WBC is often not raised in osteomyelitis in the diabetic foot.

3.5 Conservative care

Case 3.27 Good orthotic care

Not all Charcot patients benefit from surgery, and many cope well under conservative management. This was seen in the early days of the Diabetic Foot Clinic, when surgery was not an option. This case is one of a historic group of neuropaths who were treated at King's in 1979 and formed the nucleus of patients whose successful management – with a 50% reduction in amputations – led to the founding of the King's Diabetic Foot Clinic.

A 58 year old man with Type 1 diabetes of 42 years' duration and a previous history of Charcot's osteoarthropathy resulting in severe deformity of the right foot was a regular attender at the Diabetic Foot Clinic for many years. He was first seen at the age of 45 years in the Diabetic Clinic, when neuropathic ulcers of both feet were detected at a routine visit. These were Stage 3 feet. He was given bespoke shoes with cradled insoles, regular podiatry and infection control with systemic antibiotics. He worked full time as a salesman and felt unable to attend the hospital very frequently in the early years lest his sales revenues suffer from his absence. At the ages of 49 and 50 he required hospital admission for severe sepsis of the right foot, and the first, third, fourth and fifth toes were amputated when they became black from septic vasculitis. This was a Stage 5 foot.

Following the second episode of sepsis he developed acute Charcot's osteoarthropathy. He was anxious to continue working and refused to come into hospital for bedrest. This was in 1984, before the total contact casting programme had been set up. He continued to walk and developed severe deformity of the right foot (Figure 3.27a). His company became concerned about him and offered early retirement on health grounds, which was supported by the Foot Clinic and which he accepted. He was anxious to take a holiday in the South of France and complained that his hospital shoes

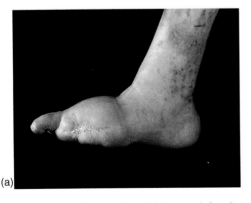
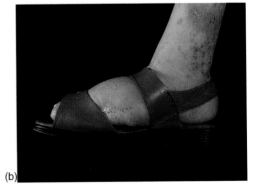

(a)   (b)

Figure 3.27   (a) Severe deformity of the right foot. (b) Special sandals.

would not be suitable. He was seen by the orthotists, and it was agreed that for short periods it would be acceptable for him to wear a pair of special sandals, which were made for him (Figure 3.27b). These had adjustable straps and cushioned insoles. Before he left he was given careful education, and advised to use a wheelchair at the airport, to check his feet very carefully every day and to refrain from sitting in the sun. He was given the telephone number of a local, English-trained chiropodist and asked to telephone the Foot Clinic if any problems arose. Nothing was heard from him until his return. The holiday had been a great success and no foot problems had developed, despite the fact that his footwear was less than optimal. He continued to attend the Foot Clinic and did well, and remained ulcer free until his death at the age of 64 from a myocardial infarct.

Learning points

- Active patients with neuropathy, a very busy lifestyle and work commitments can be difficult to manage.

- Compromise may be necessary when changes in environment render optimal footwear unsuitable.

- Holiday foot problems are very common but can often be prevented with careful education.

4

Renal Case Studies

4.1 Introduction

Diabetic patients who have kidney problems often have very special foot problems too. We see foot ulceration in a whole spectrum of diabetic patients with renal disease, ranging from low creatinine clearance to end stage renal failure treated by dialysis or renal transplantation. Renal diabetic foot problems are associated with exceedingly high rates of morbidity and mortality, and it is important to set up specialist services for these patients, who also suffer alarmingly high incidences of foot trauma and have a disconcerting propensity to develop necrosis, sometimes even in the absence of infection or vascular disease. Amputation rates are high, and the death rate is also high in renal patients, with sudden death common, and mostly due to cardiac causes.

In 1987 we realised how vulnerable these renal patients are, and we set up a Joint Renal/ Diabetic Foot Clinic at our sister hospital, Dulwich Hospital, as a satellite to the main Diabetic Foot Clinic at King's, with a view to improving outcomes in these most challenging patients. Once a month, diabetic patients with a renal transplant were seen on a Friday morning by the renal physician, and it was arranged for them also to be seen by a diabetologist and by a podiatrist for routine inspection and preventive foot care. This ensured early detection of foot problems. Diabetic patients undergoing dialysis who had foot problems also attended the dialysis centre on Friday mornings so that they could be seen. The foot outcomes of this venture were good, and when the renal transplant service moved to another London hospital, many transplant and dialysis patients continued to be seen at the main King's Diabetic Foot Clinic.

Many diabetic patients have impaired renal function, which predisposes them to foot lesions. We have also learned that infection of diabetic foot lesions can impair renal function. Patients may start off with low creatinine clearance and the infection is enough to tip them over the edge into renal failure and renal replacement therapy. Some of these patients improve when the infection has cleared and can come off dialysis, but in others the renal function never recovers and they have to stay on dialysis.

Diabetic Foot Care: Case Studies in Clinical Management   Alethea Foster and Michael Edmonds
© 2011 John Wiley & Sons, Ltd.

We also see patients with normal serum creatinine and no history of nephropathy who during episodes of severe infection develop low clearance but slowly revert to normal when infection is controlled. Reaching baseline can take six months.

It is our clear impression that all diabetic renal patients, including those with low creatinine clearance, suffer from more severe infections than other diabetic patients without renal impairment. In addition to infections with the more commonly seen micro-organisms we see devastating infections involving rarer organisms, including *Enterobacter cloacae*, *Stenotrophomonas maltophilia*, *Pseudomonas*, *Serratia*, *Citrobacter koseri* and *Streptococcus milleri*. ESBLs (extended sensitivity beta lactamases) are also a problem in renal patients. Patients with impaired renal function also deteriorate more rapidly when infected compared with neuropathic patients, and this is probably related to the impaired renal function.

Acute deterioration of renal function can be caused by dehydration as well as infection. Furthermore, deterioration can also be caused by injudicious treatment with drugs such as colchicine and non-steroidal anti-inflammatories, and several of our case histories demonstrate this. In all these patients we are very aware of the need to avoid, wherever possible, any treatment that may further damage the kidneys. For example, we use gentamicin very sparingly and only as a last resort, and always at reduced doses. Wherever possible we try to avoid the use of nephrotoxic contrast medium, and to prevent dehydration in these patients. Careful monitoring of the metabolic status is always needed, with careful choice of medications and close liaison between the Diabetic Foot Clinic and the Renal Team.

Thus diabetic foot disease develops in a spectrum of renal patients ranging from reduced glomerular filtration rate to end stage renal failure. Patients may then have a renal transplant, involving immunosuppression and a greatly increased risk of infection, or go on to haemodialysis, with fluctuating blood pressure and metabolic disturbances, or peritoneal dialysis, with risks of associated peritonitis. Whichever group they are in, diabetic patients with impaired renal function are prone to infection and rapidly become destabilised, so they are very high risk patients. A key lesson for the diabetic foot practitioner is that it is essential to be aware of the renal function of each patient.

In the early days of the renal foot clinic, our vascular surgeons were reluctant to operate on renal patients, feeling that outcomes would inevitably be very poor in patients with heavily calcified blood vessels and general frailty. However, we have recently been impressed by the results obtained by a dedicated vascular team led by Hisham Rashid in achieving successful angioplasties and bypasses in patients with end stage renal failure. During our years working with the diabetic foot, we have seen marked improvements in the management of renal patients involving angioplasty and bypass with greatly improved survival rates of both limbs and patients.

We see limited life expectancy par excellence with dialysis patients: the dialysis patient is the truly end stage renal patient and the aim in managing them is to try to improve their quality of life as much as we can. We do this by eradicating infection and getting ulcers healed as quickly as possible. We try to catch ulcers early, and heal them conservatively if possible, because invasive surgery such as amputation is not without risk for these supremely vulnerable dialysis patients.

Overall, we have described our renal patients under the following sub-headings for this chapter.

- Patients with normal serum creatinine initially who develop low creatinine clearance with infection
- Low creatinine clearance and complications
- Continuous ambulatory peritoneal dialysis (CAPD) and complications
- Haemodialysis and complications
- Renal transplant and complications
- Revascularisation in renal patients.

4.2 Patients with normal serum creatinine initially who develop low creatinine clearance with infection

Infections in the neuropathic foot are precipitated by defects in the skin caused by trauma. This may be due to chronic repetitive stress or to an acute incident, as in the following case.

Case 4.1 Vomiting and renal decompensation

A 65 year old lady, with Type 2 diabetes for 15 years, had hypertension, for which she took valsartan 160mg daily, doxazosin 8 mg daily and labetalol 400 mg daily. She had had cellulitis and was treated by her GP with flucloxacillin. He referred her to the Diabetic Foot Clinic after ten days and she was admitted with cellulitis around the left ankle. This was a Stage 4 foot. She had a serum creatinine of 78 µmol/l and eGFR of 61 ml/min. Her CRP was 36.9 mg/l, and her uric acid was normal at 0.31 mmol/l. She had a normal X-ray. An MRI showed extensive diffuse soft tissue oedema and there was prominent enhancement of Karger's fat pad (pre-Achilles). The diffuse enhancing area within Karger's fat pad and the lateral subcutaneous fat was suggestive of a cellulitis without a focal collection (Figure 4.1). She was penicillin allergic and was treated with vancomycin, and the ankle greatly improved.

After 3 days she then became nauseous, and despite treatment with anti-emetics had recurrent episodes of vomiting, with renal decompensation. She had a renal artery Duplex and there was no evidence of renal artery stenosis. A renal ultrasound showed normal kidney size, shape and position and there was no dilatation of the collecting systems. Her 24 hour urine protein was 362 mg a day (normal up to 150). She was seen by the Renal Team and they thought that she had acute tubular necrosis secondary to her nausea and vomiting. She was rehydrated and gradually improved when antihypertensive therapy was temporarily stopped. Serum creatinine rose to 159 µmol/l, and it peaked 4 days later at 299 µmol/l and then started to fall. Two weeks later, it was 182 µmol/l, and 3 months later it was 127 µmol/l with eGRF of 38 ml/min (low). Her serum creatinine only returned to normal after six months.

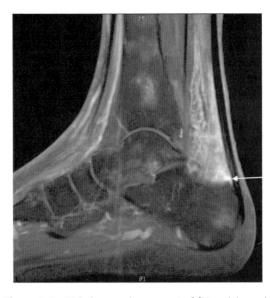

Figure 4.1   MRI shows enhancement of fat pad (arrow).

Learning points

- Diabetic patients are very vulnerable to renal damage: even with a seemingly normal serum creatinine. They are very vulnerable to decompensation if they become. dehydrated

- Diabetic patients with foot infections should have close monitoring of serum electrolytes and renal function.

- Karger's fat pad can be affected as part of soft tissue infection in the diabetic foot.

Case 4.2 Deterioration of renal function in a patient with neuropathic ulcer and infection

The next patient's foot infection put him on a path that eventually led to end stage renal failure and dialysis.

This patient was 39 years old and had Type 2 diabetes of 7 years' duration, and was insulin treated. He visited his general practitioner complaining of discomfort in his heel, and plantar fasciitis was diagnosed and treated with an injection of steroid. He developed heel ulceration (Figure 4.2), which became infected (Stage 4 foot), and he was admitted and treated with quadruple antibiotics amoxicillin 500 mg tds, flucloxacillin 500 mg qds, metronidazole 500 mg tds and ceftazidime 1 g tds. His creatinine was 96 µmol/l with eGFR of 80 ml/min and the CRP was 55.1 mg/l. X-ray showed soft tissue disruption inferior to the calcaneum.

Three months later, his foot became infected and he was admitted with a CRP of 187.5 mg/l and creatinine of 205 µmol/l. MRSA was grown and he was given IV vancomycin 1 g statim and then dosage according to serum levels. His CRP fell to 5.3 mg/l, and the creatinine to 107 µmol/l. Two years later, he was admitted under the general medical team with shortness of breath, haemoptysis and chest pain. He was hypertensive and hypoxic and had pulmonary oedema and biventricular failure. His CRP was just 5.9 mg/l. A vasculitis screen was negative. His serum creatinine had now risen to 380 µmol/l. He underwent a renal biopsy, which showed diabetic changes and some evidence of acute tubular necrosis. Eight years after initial presentation to the Foot Clinic, he was started on long-term haemodialysis.

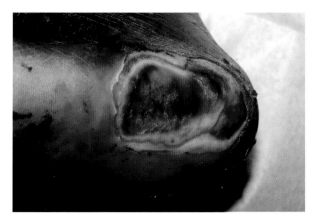

Figure 4.2 Plantar heel ulcer.

Learning points

- Diabetic patients should not have plantar injections of steroids for plantar fasciitis. Lesions of the foot provoked by steroids can easily get infected.

- We have seen several cases where steroid injection of the plantar aspect of the heel led to necrosis. In the neuropathic foot this usually responds to antibiotics and debridement. In the neuroischaemic foot, patients may need revascularisation and run the risk of amputation if this cannot be carried out.

- This patient's renal function deteriorated very quickly. He had episodes of foot infection, which may have contributed to this, although his creatinine returned to normal range on resolution of the infection.

- However, we may speculate that hypoperfusion of the kidneys during the episode of cardiac failure caused an insult from which they did not recover.

- The Diabetic Foot Clinic must be aware of these possibilities of rapid onset renal failure when treating neuropathic foot ulcers.

Case 4.3 Rapid deterioration of renal function in a patient with neuropathic feet

A 44 year old lady with Type 2 insulin treated diabetes for 8 years presented when she burnt her toes on a heater. She had two small ulcers on the apex of her left first toe. This was a Stage 3 foot. The ulcers were debrided and dressed and healed quickly. Her other complaint was of painful neuropathy in both feet and she was treated with pregabalin. She was depressed and was started on fluoxetine. She had proliferative retinopathy, which received laser photocoagulation, nephropathy, hypertension, neuropathy and diabetic diarrhoea. Interestingly, she had normal coronary vessels and normal leg vessels.

She had recurrent toe ulcers and often grew Group B *Streptococcus* and *Staphylococcus aureus*, which were treated with amoxicillin and flucloxacillin. She then became short of breath on both exertion and lying flat in bed at night and developed bilateral ankle oedema. Her echocardiogram showed the left ventricle to be mildly dilated and the left ventricular systolic function was moderately reduced. There was anterior wall and inferior wall hypokinesis. On chest X-ray she had an enlarged heart and she had a high resolution CT scan of the chest, which showed septal oedema and bilateral pleural effusions. Her ECG showed some lateral T wave invertion. A dilated cardiomyopathy was diagnosed.

Two years after initial presentation, she came to the Foot Clinic as an emergency patient. She had a puncture wound on the plantar surface of the foot, surrounded by moist, bulging skin, with cellulitis and lymphadenitis and bilateral foot oedema. This was a Stage 4 foot. She was admitted and given amoxicillin 500 mg tds, flucloxacillin 500 mg qds, metronidazole 500 mg tds and ceftazidime 1 g tds IV antibiotic therapy. Her CRP was 149.6 mg/l, with a white count of 11.56×10^9/l with neutrophils 7.94×10^9/l. Her glycated haemoglobin was 12.7%, and creatinine was 146 µmol/l. She underwent surgical drainage. The wound grew *Staphylococcus aureus* and her quadruple antibiotics were reduced to flucloxacillin when the microbiology results were known. Her serum creatinine fell to 78 µmol/l.

The following year she was admitted for uncontrolled diabetes and symptomatic hyperglycaemia and her insulin therapy was optimised. And a year later she presented with a serum creatinine of 147 µmol/l and infection of her left fifth toe, which grew *Staphylococcus aureus* and Group B *Streptococcus*. She was treated with quadruple IV antibiotics as above at first, which were then reduced to amoxicillin and flucloxacillin and serum creatinine fell to 90 µmol/l. She had a further admission in the following year for another foot infection and swelling of the left ankle, and shortly after was again admitted for shortness of breath and chest pain.

The following year, she had two further admissions. First, she was admitted with a finger pulp infection and needed a surgical drainage of the left index finger pulp and three days later needed a further drainage. Her CRP was 34.4 mg/l. Then, she was admitted for increasing shortness of breath. Her CRP was 86.4 mg/l and the creatinine had risen to 263 µmol/l. She had heart failure and pulmonary oedema. By the following year, her creatinine was 361 µmol/l and then there was a sudden rise to a creatinine of 642 µmol/l, which was caused by reduced renal perfusion secondary to new diuretic and antihypertensive therapy, which was stopped. The rise in serum creatinine was drug induced, and not related to foot infection. Over the next three months her creatinine had fallen to 365 µmol/l.

Learning points

- This was a patient with neuropathic foot disease who developed fluid retention secondary to cardiac and renal impairment.

- In each episode of foot infection, her renal function deteriorated, but with aggressive treatment of the infection it did return to within normal range after treatment.

- On developing cardiac failure, renal function decreased considerably and did not return to normal.

- There are young diabetic patients with neuropathic foot ulcers attending the Diabetic Foot Clinic who have rapid deterioration of renal function.

- Foot practitioners must be aware of this complication in order to achieve optimum multidisciplinary care.

4.3   Low creatinine clearance and complications

This group of patients already had compromised renal function when they presented to the Diabetic Foot Clinic.

Case 4.4   Low clearance in a poorly healing, non-compliant man

This patient had several episodes of foot sepsis and each one led to further renal impairment.

This 60 year old man had insulin treated Type 2 diabetes of 23 years' duration, and was known to have low creatinine clearance. He had sickle cell trait. He had neuropathy, retinopathy and nephropathy, with a creatinine of 210 µmol/l, and erectile dysfunction. He was a smoker, who continues to smoke, and worked as a taxi driver. He had attended the Diabetic Foot Clinic since 1989, developing occasional foot ulcers, and had infections with Group B *Streptococcus* and *Staphylococcus aureus*, which healed on amoxicillin and flucloxacillin taken orally. He was always very reluctant to take time off work to rest his feet, and he developed a problem ulcer at the right fifth metatarsal head. The right fifth toe had become infected (Figure 4.4a). He was admitted with a CRP of 93.9 mg/l and serum creatinine of 295 µmol/l. He was given IV quadruple antibiotics amoxicillin 500 mg tds,

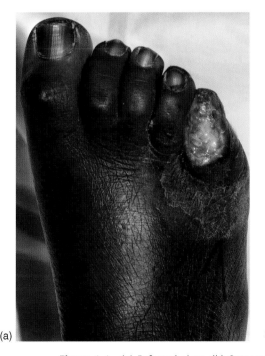
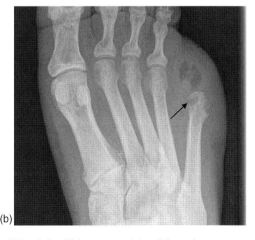

(a)   (b)

Figure 4.4   (a) Infected ulcer. (b) Osteomyelitis of the fifth metatarsal head (arrow).

flucloxacillin 500 mg qds, metronidazole 500 mg tds and ceftazidime 1 g daily and underwent surgical debridement, but insisted on an early discharge so that he could get back to
work. Serum creatinine fell to 220 μmol/l. The wound did not heal and became a chronic
ulcer.

Three months later, he was admitted for amputation of the right fifth toe and again he
was allowed to go home quite quickly. The wound had not healed when he left the hospital,
and again it developed into an indolent ulcer. Later that year, six months further on, he was
admitted for an infected ulcer under the right fifth metatarsal head. X-ray showed
osteomyelitis of the metatarsal head (Figure 4.4b). A deep swab grew mixed anaerobes
sensitive to metronidazole, *E. coli* sensitive to ceftazidime and *Serratia marcescens* sensitive
to meropenem. His serum creatinine had risen to 318 μmol/l, and CRP was 25.4 mg/l. He
was treated with IV meropenem 500 mg bd and the serum creatinine fell to 211 μmol/l.
However, he refused surgery and went home.

He deteriorated, and was readmitted two months later with serum creatinine of
288 μmol/l. He underwent debridement and fifth metatarsal head excision. He was again
given IV meropenem 500 mg bd, and serum creatinine fell to 210 μmol/l. He insisted on
early discharge after a week, but agreed to wear a total contact cast and stay at home, and
the foot healed quickly.

Learning points

- A low creatinine clearance imparts susceptibility to infection.

- This patient's serum creatinine rose during his episodes of foot infection but fell in
  response to aggressive treatment of infection.

- Episodes of infection can cause permanent renal impairment if they are not treated
  aggressively.

- Management was compromised by the patient always insisting on early discharge.

- His smoking continued despite efforts to encourage him to stop and this hindered his
  healing.

Case 4.5   Acute renal impairment after being given colchicine for gout

Deteriorating renal function may be drug related, as in this case.

This patient was 80 years old, and had Type 2 diabetes for 15 years, hypertension and myeloma. He had recurrent episodes of gout, and had had a transient ischaemic attack. His serum creatinine was 138 μmol/l with eGFR of 54 ml/min, indicating that his renal function was impaired. The patient was admitted with a hot red swollen left first metatarsophalangeal joint. X-ray showed features typical of gout, with erosions at the head of the first metatarsal (Figure 4.5). There was also a tophus on a toe on the right foot, which burst with discharge of white, chalklike material. Because the skin was broken, this was a Stage 3 foot. He had anaemia and he required two units of packed red cells. The uric acid was 0.49 mmol/l and he was given colchicine 500 micrograms bd.

After three days he developed severe diarrhoea and became dehydrated, leading to acute renal impairment. His serum creatinine was 390 μmol/l and one week later it had risen to 407 μmol/l. He was rehydrated and over the next four weeks serum creatinine gradually fell to 169 μmol/l, and the foot healed. After this acute episode of gout had resolved, he was given allopurinol and did well.

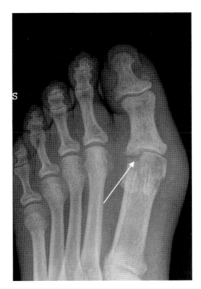

Figure 4.5   X-ray shows erosions of head of first metatarsal (arrow).

Learning points

- Diabetic patients with existing renal impairment who are treated with colchicine and develop diarrhoea can readily go into renal failure.

- Colchicine should be administered with care to diabetic patients with poor renal function.

- Colchicine should be stopped immediately if diarrhoea ensues.

Case 4.6 Optimising renal function to achieve healing of an ulcer

When patients have co-morbidities and poor renal function then foot problems can be very slow to heal.

This 58 year old lady had multiple problems including Type 2 diabetes for 15 years, peripheral neuropathy, proliferative retinopathy, diabetic nephropathy, ischaemic heart disease, hypertension, asthma, poor mobility, incontinence, morbid obesity, peripheral oedema, depression and sleep apnoea. Due to her incontinence she had a long term indwelling supra-pubic catheter. Serum creatinine was 280 μmol/l. She also had ulceration of the heel, which was very slow to heal due to her multiple co-morbidities, and it became infected with a mild degree of surrounding cellulitis. This was a Stage 4 foot and she was admitted to hospital.

She grew *Staphylococcus aureus*, *E coli* and mixed anaerobes from the heel ulcer. *E coli* was also grown from her urinary catheter. The serum creatinine had risen to 350 μmol/l. She was treated with IV meropenem 500 mg bd but with rehydration and treatment of sepsis serum creatinine fell to 295 μmol/l. The patient was anaemic and was treated with darbepoetin. She was on a low protein diet, and was started on Fortisip and also given high phosphates with Adcal. The patient was thus treated to maximise her kidney function so as to achieve healing of the ulcer. She also had sleep apnoea and respiratory problems. Overnight oximetry on room air showed 91% oxygen saturation with some evidence of hypoventilation. She had maximal treatment of nocturnal hypoventilation and reduction of peripheral oedema. Other interventions included commencement of thyroxine for newly diagnosed myxoedema. Her amitriptyline taken for depression was stopped because she became drowsy and it was aggravating her hypoventilation.

She was discharged and the ulcer healed whilst attending the Diabetic Foot Clinic. However, she was re-admitted the following year with an infected area over the right fifth metatarsal head with cellulitis (Figure 4.6). She had podiatric debridement. Tissue grew *E coli* and *Pseudomonas aeruginosa* and she was treated with IV gentamicin 120 mg statim and then dosage according to serum levels. After she went home, she was followed up in the Foot Clinic and she healed.

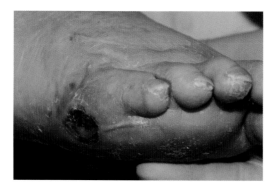

Figure 4.6   Ulcer over fifth metatarsal head.

Learning points

- In addition to treating the ulcer and any infection it is also important to optimise renal function and address any other health problems to speed healing.

- These people with low clearance and impaired renal function are on an even sharper knife edge than diabetic patients with normal renal function, and even a slight health upset such as mild infection destabilises them.

- Peripheral oedema is a potent factor in predisposing patients to ulceration and delaying healing, and should always be reduced if possible.

Case 4.7   Rapid treatment of infection can preserve kidney function

It is always important to ensure that other medical conditions are treated, instead of just focussing on the foot.

The patient was 61 years old. She was a very obese lady with Type 2 diabetes of 34 years' duration, and was originally on tablets but subsequently insulin treated. She had peripheral neuropathy. Foot pulses could not be palpated, and she had a chronic foot ulcer over the lateral aspect of the forefoot. She was noted to have renal impairment with a serum creatinine of 137 µmol/l.

The foot ulcer became infected and she was admitted immediately to hospital. A tissue sample grew *Enterobacter cloacae* sensitive to ceftazidime, gentamicin, ciprofloxacin and meropenem and *Alcaligenes faecalis* sensitive to meropenem. She was given IV meropenem 1 g bd. To ascertain the degree of ischaemia she underwent a downstream angiogram. No angioplastable lesions were seen. Her haemoglobin was 6.7 g/dl and she was transfused 3 units after surgical debridement of her ulcer and further areas of non-viable tissue on the left fourth and fifth toes and heel. The resulting wound was treated with a skin graft from a donor site on her left thigh. After two days she was started on a VAC pump and was discharged with a healing foot. Her renal function remained steady during this admission.

She deteriorated as an outpatient and needed a further admission for debridement and draining of the infected left foot ulcer. Her serum creatinine rose to 144 µmol/l, falling to 125 µmol/l by two months later. She continued to visit her local hospital.

Learning points

- Prompt treatment of infection in diabetic foot patients can preserve kidney function. In her first admission renal function remained stable, and during her second admission there was only a small rise in serum creatinine, which resolved.

- Often, diabetic foot infections are polymicrobial and need accurate antibiotic treatment.

- It is not possible to guess the bacteria on these wounds and it is preferable to send infected tissue for culture.

- If the clinician is in doubt as to the degree of ischaemia, then an angiogram should be performed.

Case 4.8   Holiday foot trauma and an apparently minor foot problem acted as a portal of entry for infection leading to acute renal failure

Any break in the skin, no matter how small, can be a portal of entry for devastating infection.

A 32 year old lady with Type 1 diabetes since the age of 2 years, hypothyroidism, diabetic retinopathy, history of transient ischaemic attack, hypertension, diabetic nephropathy and chronic kidney disease with impaired renal function (serum creatinine 126 μmol/l) was abroad on holiday in the Maldives. She went into the sea and was stung by a jellyfish between her toes. The next day she began to feel unwell and decided to fly home early. En route her condition deteriorated, she started vomiting and her family brought her to the hospital straight from the airport. She was ketotic and very unwell, with a low BP of 60/40 mm Hg, and was admitted to the Intensive Care Unit. She rapidly went into acute on chronic renal failure and had to be haemodialysed.

She was at first thought to have a urinary tract infection. However, the Diabetic Foot Team was asked to see her. It was noted that she had interdigital necrosis at the site of the sting, which nevertheless appeared to be very superficial with minimal cellulitis (Figure 4.8a, b). A wound swab was taken. Group A *Streptococcus* was grown from the wound swab and also from two blood cultures taken on admission. She was given IV clindamycin 600 mg qds and high doses of benzyl penicillin 2.4 g qds, and total parenteral nutrition (TPN). When in the Intensive Care Unit she had some sudden episodes of hypotension followed by bradycardia. They occurred without warning. The sudden onset reflected cardiovascular instability in a patient with severe autonomic neuropathy. These hypotensive episodes were treated with fluid boluses. She was discharged to the ward after 11 days, was able to come off dialysis and made a complete recovery.

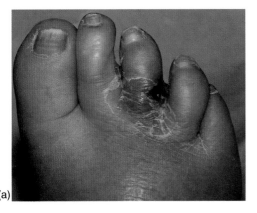

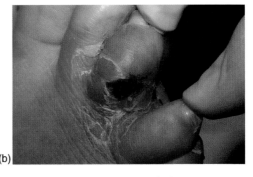

(a)   (b)

Figure 4.8   (a) Forefoot with interdigital ulcer. (b) Close-up of interdigital ulcer.

Learning points

- Group A *Streptococcus* can complicate even a very small injury to the foot. An apparently minor foot problem can be a portal of entry for severe sepsis, as in this case.

- Bacteraemia can lead to a rapid deterioration of renal function in diabetic patients.

- Diabetic patients with autonomic neuropathy and nephropathy have lost their homeostatic reflexes and become very unstable, as regards the cardiovascular system, if they develop a systemic illness such as a bacteraemia. This often manifests itself as episodes of hypotension.

Case 4.9 Patient who went on to dialysis because of sepsis

Foot infection was the cause of this patient's deteriorating renal function.

This 60 year old man with Type 2 diabetes, ulcerative colitis with ileostomy and diabetic nephropathy was attending the low creatinine clearance clinic and was thought to be rapidly approaching end stage renal failure. He had had an elective admission for the formation of a left radiocephalic fistula in preparation for dialysis. His creatinine was 490 μmol/l and his eGFR was 11 ml/min. Two months later, the patient was transferred to the Renal Ward at King's with deteriorating renal function, having been admitted to his local hospital with a gangrenous right big toe (Stage 5 foot). Amputation of the right hallux and two further surgical debridements had already been performed at his local hospital. This was now a Stage 4 foot. His CRP was 91.2 mg/l, with WBC of 14.14×10^9/l of which 12.28×10^9/l were neutrophils. Swabs taken from the foot grew *Klebsiella pneumoniae*, *Enterobacter cloacae*, mixed anaerobes and *Enterococcus faecalis*. He was first treated with quadruple IV antibiotics amoxicillin 500 mg tds, flucloxacillin 500 mg qds, metronidazole 500 mg tds and ceftazidime 500 mg od and then with IV meropenem 500 mg od. On admission to King's the serum creatinine was 471 μmol/l, and it fell to 354 μmol/l and he did not need dialysis. Foot pulses were not palpable, and an angiogram was carried out and demonstrated no significant femoral popliteal disease, normal trifurcation below the knee and three vessel straight line run off to the ankle supplying the foot. He was discharged with a healing wound, which was treated locally and did well.

The next year he developed infection of his left heel (Figure 4.9a) and was admitted with a CRP of 64.9 mg/l and serum creatinine of 629 μmol/l. He had hyperkalaemia and acidosis and was haemodialysed as an emergency. He had a Duplex angiogram showing triphasic flow at the left ankle and no significant femoral or popliteal disease. MRSA was grown from the foot and he was treated with IV vancomycin 1 g statim and then dosage according to

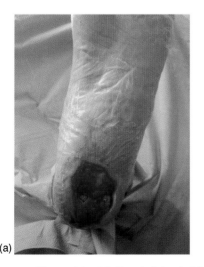

(a)

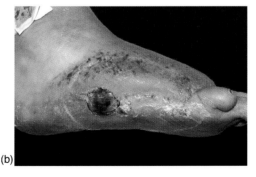

(b)

Figure 4.9 (a) Ulcer left heel. (b) Original right foot lesion has almost healed.

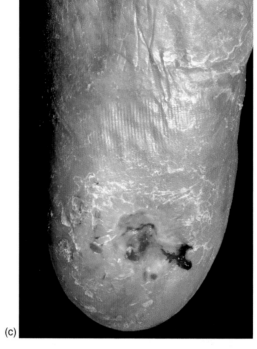

(c)

Figure 4.9 *(continued)*   (c) Left heel is healing.

serum levels. The patient also had a PICC line inserted and multiple debridements on the ward, and a VAC pump was applied. Although the infection was controlled, the renal function did not improve and he remained on haemodialysis. He received shared care from the Diabetic Foot Clinic at King's and his local district nursing service, community podiatry service and local hospital, including very regular checks of his feet. The original right foot lesion has almost healed (Figure 4.9b); the left heel is healing under treatment (Figure 4.9c).

Learning points

- Diabetic patients with low creatinine clearance are very susceptible to ulceration, which often becomes complicated by polymicrobial infection, including Gram negative infections.

- Although renal function deteriorated during the patient's infection of the right foot, it subsequently improved and he avoided haemodialysis.

- However, during the infection of the left heel, renal function was impaired to a life threatening situation and the patient had to remain on dialysis.

- When treating diabetic foot infections in patients with low creatinine clearance, it is important to be aware that renal function may deteriorate rapidly and the patient may urgently need some form of renal replacement therapy.

Case 4.10 Low clearance followed by acute destabilisation needing temporary dialysis

When patients develop renal failure during a health crisis they may require dialysis for a short time only, as in this case.

This patient developed Charcot foot with a rocker bottom deformity complicated by neuropathic ulceration (Figure 4.10). This was a Stage 3 foot. He was seen by the orthopaedic surgeons and it was decided to perform an exostectomy to promote healing of the ulcer. The patient had hypertension, which was treated with amlodipine, and he also took ramipril. Preoperatively, the blood pressure was between 140 and 150 mm Hg systolic over 80 to 90 mm Hg diastolic. The preoperative eGFR was 23 ml/min, the serum creatinine 260 µmol/l, haemoglobin 12.4 g/dl, CRP 62.9 mg/l. The patient was admitted to hospital and underwent exostectomy (Figure 4.10). The blood pressure was low

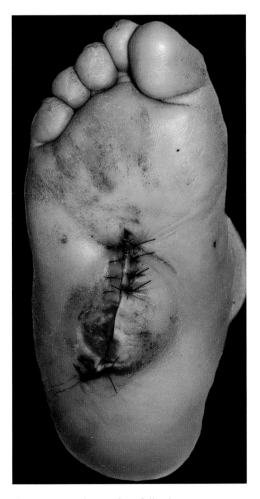

Figure 4.10 Charcot foot following exostectomy.

during the operation, being 90/60 mm Hg, but this recovered postoperatively to 120/80 mm Hg. On the second postoperative day, the patient collapsed whilst standing upright and was thought to have had a postural hypotensive episode. However, the patient had raised serum troponin at 0.66 μg/l and inverted T waves over the anteroseptal chest leads. Urine output was low, at less than 30 ml/min. Serum creatinine had risen to 303 μmol/l and the following day was 385 μmol/l with urea 18.8 mmol/L, albumin 29 g/l, bicarbonate 23 mmol/l and haemoglobin 8.3 g/dl.

Three days postoperatively the serum creatinine had risen to 385 μmol/l. Initially the patient had been continued on the antihypertensive medication but this was then stopped. The serum creatinine continued to rise, and six days postoperatively reached 475 μmol/l and the patient underwent haemodialysis. His renal function recovered to its baseline value and he did not need permanent dialysis.

Learning points

- Patients with low clearance are susceptible to haemodynamic disturbances perioperatively.

- Patients who have hypotension need very close observation and their existing anti-hypertensives may need to be temporarily withdrawn.

- Very close monitoring of their renal function perioperatively is necessary.

- Patients with a low clearance can rapidly proceed to life threatening renal failure.

Case 4.11   Patient destabilised by non-steroidals

This case was destabilised when she was given pain relief, but her creatinine later returned to normal.

   This 75 year old diabetic lady with Type 2 diabetes, diagnosed 10 years previously and insulin requiring, had hypertension and chronic renal failure (baseline serum creatinine was 145 µmol/l with an eGFR of 44 ml/min). She had been admitted to hospital as an emergency, because of a fall. Whilst on the ward she was noted to have infected foot ulceration, which was painful, and she was treated by the on-call team with non-steroidal anti-inflammatories. She had good foot perfusion and all peripheral pulses were well felt. A Doppler study showed triphasic flow in the pedal vessels both sides. Her baseline creatinine was 145 µmol/l. No new medication was started except diclofenac at 50 mg bd, which was given for three days and then stopped, and clarithromycin 500 mg bd for the foot infection.

   Her serum creatinine rose to 257 µmol/l. She became short of breath with scattered crepitations in the chest and developed peripheral oedema. A diagnosis of cardiac failure and renal failure was made following her course of non-steroidal anti-inflammatories. Her oxygen saturation was 82% on air. The patient was given frusemide 40 mg daily. She had mild to moderate left ventricular systolic dysfunction on echocardiogram. Autoantibody screen was negative. There were normal serum immunoglobulins and no paraproteins, ruling out myeloma. Ultrasound of the kidneys showed a non-dilated system, and four weeks later her serum creatinine was 135 µmol/l.

Learning points

- Non-steroidal anti-inflammatory drugs can cause major problems in diabetic patients with low creatinine clearance.

- Renal function can be acutely impaired by a single dose of non-steroidal anti-inflammatory drugs, leading to severe fluid retention. This can lead to right and left ventricular failure.

4.4   Continuous ambulatory peritoneal dialysis (CAPD) and complications

We now describe several cases of foot disease in patients with end stage renal failure treated with CAPD. It is our impression that these patients are very susceptible to infection, proceed very rapidly to necrosis, and have a poorer outlook than those on haemodialysis.

Case 4.12   Post-amputation infected wound and angioplasty

A 61 year old lady, with Type 1 diabetes for 32 years, had retinopathy and end stage nephropathy and was always very prone to hypoglycaemia. She had been admitted for insertion of a peritoneal dialysis catheter and started CAPD. She had an infected ulcer on her right first toe, from which anaerobic *Streptococcus* was grown, and she was treated with oral metronidazole 400 mg tds. This was a Stage 4 foot but the infection responded to metronidazole therapy.

One year later, she underwent angiography because of persistent ulceration. Narrowing was noted within both common iliacs next to the origin. On the right the external iliac, superficial femoral artery and profunda were relatively disease free. The popliteal was normal. There was, however, narrowing of the anterior tibial and at the origin of the peroneal and posterior tibial. On the left there was narrowing within the anterior tibial peroneal and posterior tibial. Initially she had a balloon angioplasty of the right common iliac followed by a stent inserted into the right common iliac artery. One month later, she had balloon angioplasty of the right anterior tibial at three sites and the proximal peroneal artery at two sites.

Two months later, she had a further episode of infection of the right first toe, with MRSA and *E. coli* isolated, and she was treated with IV gentamicin 120 mg and vancomycin 1 g both statim and then dosages according to serum levels. She underwent repeat angioplasty of the right anterior tibial artery, tibioperoneal trunk and peroneal arteries using a 4 mm balloon and she also had an angioplasty to the origin of the posterior tibial artery with a 3 mm balloon.

Three months later, she was admitted again with an infected right first toe with a CRP of 84.6 mg/l and WBC of 11.99×10^9/l and her creatinine was 402 μmol/l. She was offered a right first toe amputation, but refused. She responded again to IV antibiotics.

The following year she had a series of hospital admissions. She had an infected left great toe. Wound swabs grew *Klebsiella* and MRSA. She was given gentamicin and vancomycin. Then she presented with right sided weakness and a CT scan showed an infarct in the left parietal lobe. A month later she had a further episode of sepsis of the left great toe and grew *Alcaligenes xylosoxidans* sensitive to meropenem from the foot. She also grew *Enterococcus faecalis* and *Pseudomonas* species. In three further episodes she was transferred from her local hospital once having had a severe hypoglycaemic episode. She was admitted with peritonitis and treated with vancomycin and gentamicin and re-admitted after having a major convulsion in hypoglycaemia. She had a long previous history of developing "hypos" without warning.

The following year she presented with an infected wound in the left foot after an amputation of the second to fifth lesser toes five weeks previously at her local hospital. She had deep sloughy ulcers with a communicating tract to exposed bone (Figure 4.12a).

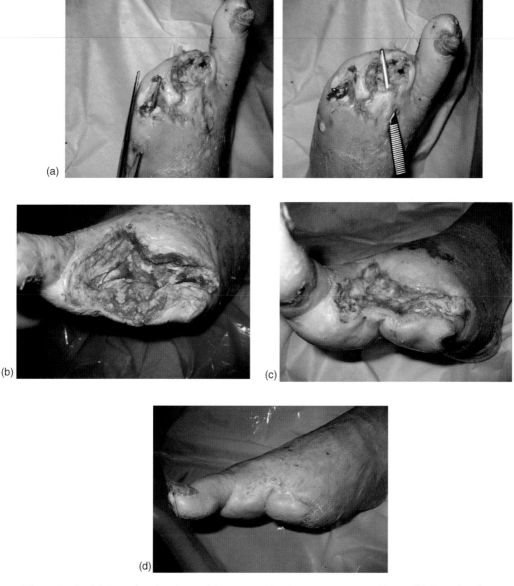

Figure 4.12 (a) Deep sloughy ulcers with a communicating tract to exposed bone. (b) Wound 24 hours post-operatively. (c) Wound after 4 weeks VAC therapy. (d) Healed wound.

A wound swab grew MRSA and she was treated with vancomycin. She had a tight stenosis in the left mid superficial femoral artery. There was narrowing of the popliteal and stenosis of the anterior tibial, posterior tibial and peroneal arteries at their origins. The superficial femoral artery was dilated with a 6 mm balloon and a 2 mm balloon was used to dilate all three vessels at the trifurcation, and she underwent surgical debridement of non-viable tissue and bone. She commenced VAC therapy 24 hours post-operatively (Figure 4.12b). She had VAC therapy for seven weeks (Figure 4.12c) and eventually healed after 16 weeks (Figure 4.12d).

Learning points

- Diabetic foot patients on peritoneal dialysis are very prone to sepsis.

- This may take the form of recurrent foot ulceration and sepsis.

- However, diabetic patients on peritoneal dialysis are also very prone to peritonitis and line infections.

- Infecting organisms in renal patients can range from classical gram positive organisms to unusual gram negatives such as *Alcaligenes xylosoxidans*.

- VAC therapy is very helpful in treating post-operative wounds in patients on dialysis.

- Diabetic patients on peritoneal dialysis are extremely frail and vulnerable patients needing close follow-up in the Diabetic Foot Clinic.

Case 4.13 Infection, necrosis and Charcot foot

This patient had a pair of "end stage" diabetic renal feet.

This 50 year old man had Type 1 diabetes of 18 years' duration. He had proliferative retinopathy and was blind in the left eye. He had mild aortic stenosis and left ventricular hypertrophy. He had hyperlipidaemia, hypertension, sensory neuropathy and end stage renal failure, treated with CAPD. He had undergone a parathyroidectomy because he had calciphylaxis (calcium deposits in skin leading to ulceration) of both legs. He had also developed necrosis of two of his fingers. He was referred to King's, with a right foot ulcer, cellulitis and necrotic right second, third and fourth toes. This was a Stage 5 foot with an MRSA infection. He was admitted and treated with IV vancomycin 1 g statim and then dosage according to serum levels. The necrotic toes were amputated. After discharge. he was treated with IV teicoplanin 200 mg three times weekly and was followed at King's Diabetic Foot Clinic. The foot did not heal and three months later he developed necrosis of the right first and fifth toes. He then noticed that his foot was changing shape (Figure 4.13a) and was admitted with infected necrotic lesions on the right foot and a right Charcot ankle. An MRI

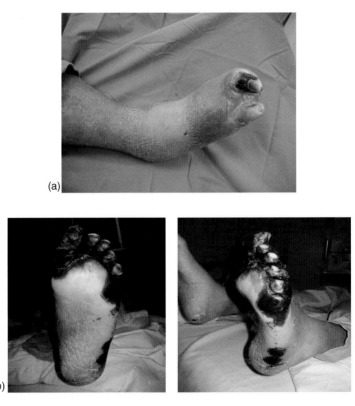

Figure 4.13 (a) Shape change at right ankle. (b) Necrotic left foot.

revealed there was a 5 cm × 3 cm × 2 cm abscess in the plantar soft tissue of the foot at the level of the metatarsal bases. He underwent surgical debridement and drainage and he was treated with vancomycin 1 g in his dialysis bags, to which his MRSA infection responded. His Charcot ankle was then treated with a total contact cast.

Eighteen months later he developed extensive dry necrosis of the left foot (Figure 4.13b) and was admitted for left leg angiogram and angioplasty. He had eccentric plaque in the above knee popliteal artery and he had some narrowing of the proximal anterior tibial. He had tight stenosis at the origin of the tibial peroneal trunk. There was a proximal stenosis of the peroneal, and in the posterior tibial there was virtual occlusion over the first centimetre. The popliteal was angioplastied and also the proximal anterior tibial artery, posterior tibial trunk, peroneal artery and posterior tibial artery. He initially improved, but six weeks later was admitted with very extensive left mid-foot plantar necrosis and forefoot necrosis and had a left below knee amputation.

His right Charcot ankle had been treated in a total contact cast for two years, but despite this treatment he had a cavovarus fixed deformity with a 90° marked varus deformity at the right ankle joint. The talus was dislocated and rotated through 90° on the AP view. For him it was a very precious foot, since without it he would be a bilateral major amputee and lose independence. He had a Taylor Spatial Frame applied to the right foot. One month later, he became unwell and septic. Two sources of sepsis were detected. He had a septic arthritis of the right knee and pus cells were obtained from aspirated joint fluid. Gram negative rods were also isolated from the peritoneal dialysis fluid. He was treated with IV meropenem 500 mg od and IV vancomycin and responded well.

Two months later, he underwent internal fixation with a nail through the heel to internally stabilise his right Charcot ankle. In the 12 hour postoperative period he had a respiratory arrest. His ventilation was assisted through a facial mask and he recovered well. Otherwise he made a good postoperative recovery. *Klebsiella pneumoniae* sensitive to meropenem was cultured from the foot wounds but the foot wounds looked healthy after IV meropenem therapy. However, ten days later he became septic. *Candida parapsilosis* was grown from blood culture bottles and he was treated with anti fungal therapy, but failed to respond and died.

Learning points

- This patient illustrates the multiple problems of diabetic patients with end stage renal failure on peritoneal dialysis.

- These patients are particularly prone to the development of. necrosis.

- Such necrosis may be precipitated by infection but is often spontaneous. It often occurs in patients who have developed digital necrosis of fingers.

- Diabetic renal patients are also prone to *Candida* infections.

- It is important to look for distal arterial disease in patients on peritoneal dialysis, including those who have traditionally been regarded as neuropathic patients.

Case 4.14 Multiple complications of diabetes and comorbidities in a CAPD patient

The development of necrotic fingers is an ominous sign in renal patients. This case was a man with multiple problems including very painful necrosis involving the fingers, and numerous episodes of sepsis.

This man was 50 years old with Type 1 diabetes. In the past he had laser photocoagulation treatment for retinopathy. His renal biopsy showed nephropathy and IgA positive crescents. He had severe neuropathy. He had bicuspid aortic stenosis and had a mechanical aortic valve replacement with long term warfarin therapy. He had a pacemaker inserted. His coronary angiogram showed normal coronary arteries. He had a supra-pubic catheter for a neuropathic bladder. He was initially admitted on to the renal ward with fluid overload and infected venous stasis ulcers. Initially he had haemodialysis, and was treated with piperacillin–tazobactam, flucloxacillin, vancomycin and gentamicin. A peritoneal dialysis catheter was inserted, and he started peritoneal dialysis. He also had a penile infection with E coli treated with meropenem and yeasts in the urine treated with fluconazole.

He was then admitted with infected ulceration of the second and fourth toes. E. coli was grown from tissue. He had a raised CRP of 129.6 mg/l and WBC 10.75×10^9/l with 8.51×10^9/l neutrophils (slightly raised). He was given IV meropenem 500 mg od and amikacin 7.5 mg/kg with re-dosing when serum level was less than 5 mg/l. He initially responded but four weeks later was admitted with infected gangrenous toes of the right foot, specifically involving the second and fourth toes. This was a Stage 5 foot. He had surgical debridement of a plantar sinus and amputation of the middle three toes of the right foot (Figure 4.14a). The tissue grew Pseudomonas aeruginosa sensitive to amikacin and gentamicin and resistant to meropenem and Serratia marcescens sensitive to ceftazidime, gentamicin and meropenem, and he was given IV gentamicin 120 mg statim and then according to serum levels.

Later that year, he was admitted because of subdural haematomas following a fall. It was decided to treat them conservatively. His warfarin dose was reduced but not stopped because of his mechanical aortic valve. By this time, he had significant distal necrosis affecting all the fingertips but specifically severe on the right ring finger, where it extended circumferentially up to the metacarpalphalangeal joint. This was associated with swelling and pain (Figure 4.14b). His INR was within the target range of 3.4. A full vasculitic screen, including cryoglobulins, was negative.

This was followed by two further admissions with severely necrotic feet over the subsequent three months. He had foot inflammation and necrosis and was still growing E coli, which was an ESBL producer sensitive to meropenem and resistant to ceftazidime and piperacillin/tazobactam, and he was prescribed IV meropenem (Figure 4.14c). His second admission was precipitated by unresolved wet necrosis of both feet. Angiography showed no significant iliac or femoral artery disease and an anterior tibial artery and posterior tibial artery straight line run to the ankle and foot. The foot cultures grew Pseudomonas aeruginosa sensitive to tobramycin and E coli sensitive to amikacin and meropenem, and he was treated with IV

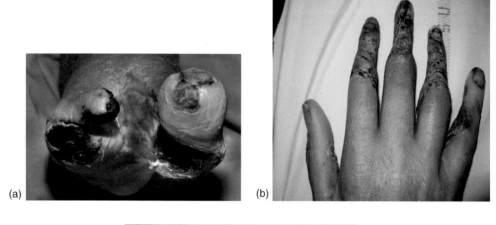

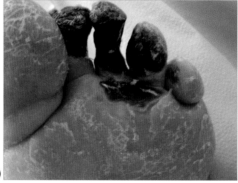

Figure 4.14 (a) Amputation of the middle three toes of the right foot. (b) Necrotic fingers, which were very painful. (c) Digital necrosis left foot.

amikacin and meropenem. He later grew a vancomycin resistant *Enteroccocum faecium* IV and was treated with linezolid 600 mg bd.

In view of his recurrent admissions for extensive necrosis it was decided to go for an elective left below knee amputation. Post-operative recovery was difficult and his overall condition deteriorated. He was semiconscious with few lucid moments, though generally drowsy and hypotensive despite fluid replacement. The amputation stump developed extensive necrosis and became very painful. The decision was made to switch to palliative care, in particular to relieve his pain, and he died.

Learning points

- Spontaneous digital necrosis in hands seems to be a marker of susceptibility to spontaneous necrosis elsewhere in the body, particularly the lower limbs.

- The cause of this spontaneous necrosis is unknown.

- Necrosis in the lower limbs was not related to macrovascular disease, as the peripheral angiogram was normal.

- Secondary infection of necrotic lesions of the feet is a major problem in these patients, with ever increasingly resistant gram negative organisms isolated.

- Throughout his treatment he was anxious to continue with active treatment, including antibiotics.

- We were criticised for the repeated admissions and it was thought that major amputation was indicated. In the event, it was not a panacea!

4.5 Haemodialysis and complications

The next group of cases covers patients treated with haemodialysis for their end stage renal failure.

Case 4.15   Diabetes, comorbidity and mortality

This lady needed amputation of all the toes on her left foot, followed by a transmetatarsal amputation.

This lady was 84 year old and had Type 2 diabetes for 15 years. She also had ischaemic heart disease with atrial fibrillation. She was on haemodialysis and developed an infection of the left foot with necrosis and was referred to King's after she had had a minor amputation locally (Figure 4.15a). Her CRP was 328 mg/l and her white count was 17.7×10^9/l, with 15.74×10^9/l neutrophils. She was initially treated with IV amoxicillin 500 mg tds, flucloxacillin 500 mg qds, metronidazole 500 mg tds and ceftazidime 500 mg od. A wound swab grew mixed anaerobes, and she was then treated with IV metronidazole. X-ray revealed multiple locules of gas within the soft tissues of the left forefoot with soft tissue swelling. There was bone destruction with loss of cortex of the distal metatarsal of the second and third left toes. There was destruction of the metatarsophalangeal joint of the third toe.

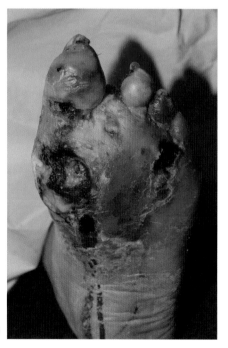
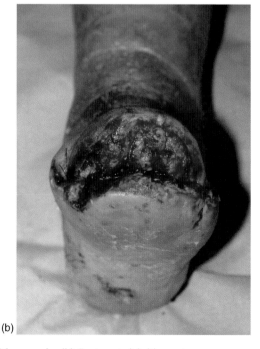

(a)   (b)

Figure 4.15   (a) Infected left foot with necrosis. (b) Foot post debridement.

Duplex scan showed triphasic pulsatile flow in the femoral and popliteal arteries. The peroneal artery was patent to mid-calf level, and the anterior tibial artery and the posterior tibial arteries were patent throughout the calf. She had amputation of the left first and second toes and then transmetatarsal amputation (Figure 4.15b). She received VAC therapy and after discharge was followed as an outpatient in the Diabetic Foot Clinic and eventually healed.

Learning points

- Infection can spread rapidly though the foot of a diabetic patient on haemodialysis and lead to extensive wet necrosis.

- Necrosis must be removed surgically and urgently: the renal diabetic foot does not tolerate wet necrosis well.

- A patient on dialysis will deteriorate systemically in the presence of foot sepsis and necrosis.

- The peripheral circulation should be addressed. In this case there was already existing straight line flow to the foot.

- Foot infection should be treated aggressively to prevent deterioration in renal function.

- VAC therapy is especially useful in the treatment of postoperative wounds in the diabetic patient in end stage renal failure.

Case 4.16   Infection and digital necrosis in a haemodialysis patient

A 50 year old lady with Type 1 diabetes for 26 years who was on haemodialysis developed digital necrosis of the first and fifth toes of the left foot and was referred to the Diabetic Foot Clinic. She had several admissions for sepsis before the toes were amputated. She underwent angiography. The peroneal artery was patent to mid-calf but then occluded. The posterior tibial artery occluded at its origin, but the anterior tibial artery went to the ankle and there was a mid-level stenosis, which was balloon dilated to 3 mm. The first and fifth toes were then amputated (Figure 4.16a, b) and she underwent VAC therapy (Figure 4.16c) and the foot healed (Figure 4.16d).

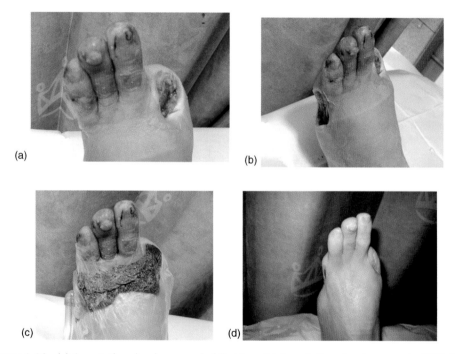

(a)   (b)

(c)   (d)

Figure 4.16   (a) Amputation showing wound of first toe. (b) Amputation showing wound of fifth toe. (c) VAC therapy. (d) Healed foot.

Learning points

- Digital necrosis in the renal ischaemic foot can be treated by minor amputation followed by VAC therapy to accelerate wound healing.

- It is all to the better if the peripheral circulation can be improved by angioplasty as in this case.

- However, in cases where the circulation cannot be improved the use of VAC therapy has usually allowed satisfactory healing to be achieved.

- Before the advent of VAC therapy these toes were often left and allowed to auto-amputate, but it was always difficult to achieve autoamputation of the first toe, and we only achieved 50% healing. Autoamputation of the lesser toes was more successful but took many months.

4.6 Renal transplant and complications

Outcomes are usually better in transplant patients than in dialysis patients, and amputations can often be avoided.

Case 4.17 A patient who prefers amputation to taking antibiotics

In the following case the patient underwent partial amputation of several toes. . . by her own choice.

This lady was first seen at the Diabetic Foot Clinic as a very irregularly attending neuropathic patient, who had good foot pulses but had recurrent foot ulceration and a great aversion to wearing hospital shoes. She was 50 years old and had Type 1 diabetes for 34 years. She had diabetic nephropathy leading to end stage renal failure and commenced haemodialysis, then moving on to CAPD for 3 years before receiving a renal transplant and long term immunosuppression.

She had frequent episodes of neuropathic ulceration with late presentations to the Diabetic Foot Clinic. She was seen by the orthopaedic surgeon for persisting ulceration of the apex of the right second toe, and underwent a partial amputation for MRSA osteomyelitis in a Stage 4 foot. Three years later, she had distal phalanx amputation of the right third toe, again for osteomyelitis, and since then has had recurrent foot ulcerations requiring rapid antibiotic treatment, particularly on the tips of her left second and third toes. In the two subsequent years, she underwent amputation of the terminal phalanx of her left third and second toes. She does not tolerate antibiotics and says that she prefers having a partial toe amputation to taking antibiotics long term.

Learning points

- Although renal transplant patients are fitter than patients on dialysis, they still encounter problems with long term immunosuppression.

- Often, long term antibiotics are needed to heal foot ulcers in these patients, some of whom may not tolerate this.

- This lady could not take oral antibiotics. She was able to tolerate short courses of parenteral antibiotics.

- She elected to undergo digital amputations rather than have long term conservative therapy.

- She preferred to have definitive surgical treatment to avoid severe spreading infections on immunosuppression that may endanger her limb, her transplanted kidney and her life.

Case 4.18   A new lease of life following elective surgery

This renal transplant patient had no serious foot problems until he developed pain in his right foot. All diabetic patients need rapid access to a foot clinic if pain arises.

A 43 year old man with Type 1 diabetes of 28 years' duration had proliferative retinopathy treated with laser photocoagulation, and end stage-renal failure due to diabetic nephropathy treated by renal transplant. He had previously undergone amputation of the first toe for osteomyelitis at another hospital and was then referred to the King's Diabetic Foot Clinic for follow-up care. He arrived in a wheelchair, accompanied by his wife. Their complaint was that if he walked more than a few steps in his current footwear his foot became blistered. His VPT was 45 V, and his pedal pulses were palpable.

There was a prominent sesamoid over the first metatarsophalangeal joint, and the adjoining skin was blistered (Figure 4.18a). This was a Stage 3 foot. The podiatrist debrided and de-roofed the blistered area, which connected with an area of callus over the first metatarsophalangeal joint (Figure 4.18b, c) to expose a neuropathic ulcer (Figure 4.18d). Despite regular debridements and provision of new shoes with cradled insoles, the patient continued to develop callus and ulceration unless he used a wheelchair. He became very upset and frustrated by the limitations on his activities, particularly since he was a keen golf player and had recently purchased a timeshare apartment in Florida near a golf course.

He was referred to the orthopaedic surgeon for a procedure to excise the prominent sesamoid and smooth off the metatarsal head. He was given prophylactic antibiotics amoxicillin 500 mg tds and flucloxacillin 500 mg qds because of the immunosuppression (cyclosporine A, azathioprine and prednisolone), which predisposed him to infection. He healed in four weeks, was fitted with new insoles, was followed long-term in the Diabetic Foot Clinic and remained ulcer-free. He plays golf regularly and makes regular trips to his holiday home. "Life is good again", he said.

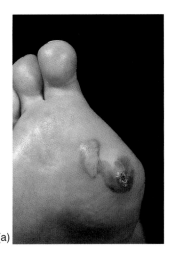
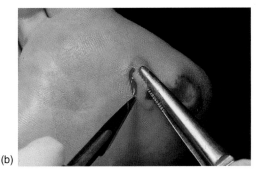

(a)   (b)

Figure 4.18   (a) Prominent sesamoid over the first metatarsophalangeal joint, and blistered adjoining skin. (b) Debriding the blistered area.

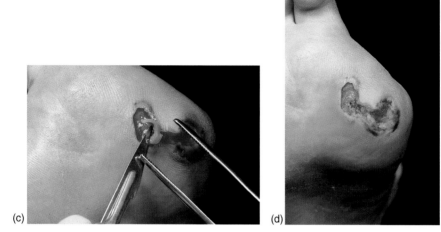

Figure 4.18 (*continued*)   (c) Debriding and de-roofing the blistered area. (d) Neuropathic ulcer.

Learning points

- An underlying bony prominence on the plantar surface creates an area of high pressure, which is prone to develop callus and to ulcerate. In this case, the effects on the patient's life were considerable. He was a young man who resented having to use a wheelchair.

- Outcomes in the renal foot can be very good, especially in renal transplant patients, if care is meticulous.

- Surgery alone is not always the solution. Good footwear will also be needed.

Case 4.19   Iatrogenic necrosis

We previously described a case of necrosis developing after a capillary blood sample was taken from a foot. In the next case, necrosis developed after an IV line was inserted into the foot of a diabetic patient with a renal transplant.

A 59 year old man, with Type 2 diabetes of 9 years' duration, peripheral neuropathy with VPT above 50 V, palpable pedal pulses, proliferative retinopathy treated with laser photocoagulation and end stage renal failure due to diabetic nephropathy treated with cadaveric renal transplant, was brought to Casualty after collapsing at home after an episode of diarrhoea and vomiting. He was hypotensive. An IV line was inserted into one of his dorsal foot veins after attempts to use arm veins had failed and he received IV fluids, which inadvertently went subcutaneously.

Three days later a patch of discolouration was noted on the dorsum of the foot. This became an area of deep necrosis (Figure 4.19), which healed after five months during which time he rested and elevated the foot as much as possible, received daily dressings and inspections from the District Nursing Service, and attended the Diabetic Foot Clinic at weekly intervals.

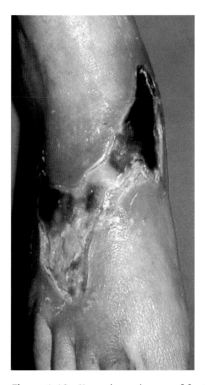

Figure 4.19 Necrosis on dorsum of foot.

Learning points

- Any injury to the feet of a high-risk patient is best avoided and foot veins should never be used for vascular access.

- A traumatic wound is liable to develop necrosis in renal feet, even in the absence of infection or ischaemia.

- Necrotic lesions following trauma in a well perfused renal foot may have a good outcome with optimal care.

4.7   Revascularisation in renal patients

Although we have emphasized the fragility of renal patients with neuroischaemic feet, our experience is that they respond very well to revascularisation.

Case 4.20   A patient on dialysis with multiple comorbidities who has a successful bypass

This 76 year old man had insulin-treated Type 2 diabetes for 32 years, and had been on haemodialysis for 8 years for end stage renal failure from diabetic nephropathy. He had a previous history of CVA, hypertension and proliferative retinopathy, with surgery to the right eye for vitreous haemorrhage. He had right hemicolectomy for ischaemic bowel. He also had vascular dementia. He was seen in the Diabetic Foot Clinic with necrosis of the right first toe. This was a Stage 5 foot. He was started on aspirin and statin. A wound swab grew *Staphylococcus aureus*. He was treated with vancomycin 1 g statim and then dosage according to serum levels. An angiogram showed disease at the trifurcation (Figure 4.20a) with reconstitution of the anterior tibial artery on the right side (Figure 4.20b). He underwent angioplasty of the trifurcation.

The necrosis of the right first toe of the patient worsened and the toe then grew *Serratia marcescens* sensitive to ciprofloxacin and gentamicin. He had a right popliteal to anterior tibial artery bypass and right toe amputation. He had larva therapy, followed by VAC therapy. Throughout his time with us he was given his antibiotics through his haemodialysis and was given vancomycin and gentamicin. He has weekly review by the Diabetic Foot Team when he has his dialysis. The arterial graft is functioning perfectly with a good triphasic signal and the right foot has healed well.

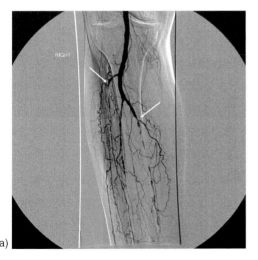
(a)

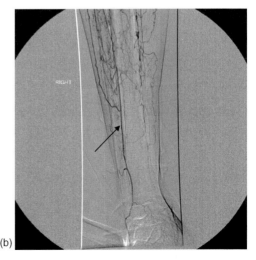
(b)

Figure 4.20   (a) Disease at the trifurcation (arrows). (b) Reconstitution of the anterior tibial artery (arrow).

Learning points

- Although angioplasty improved the perfusion to the foot, it did not return pulsatile blood flow.

- Successful distal arterial bypasses are able to provide pulsatile blood flow and are possible despite end stage renal failure and multiple co-morbidities.

- For the future wellbeing of the patient, much will depend on regular graft surveillance and servicing of grafts.

Case 4.21 Successful bypass despite multiple comorbidities

Even the presence of multiple comorbidities need not preclude revascularisation.

A man with Type 2 diabetes and multiple problems, including a history of hyperparathyroidism, end stage renal failure treated with haemodialysis, hypertension, hyperlipidaemia, sclerodema of Buschke, blindness due to diabetic retinopathy, an upper gastro-intestinal bleed from a moderate haemorrhagic gastritis and a benign looking fundal polyp, developed wet necrosis of his right first toe and was admitted. This was a Stage 5 foot. He was given IV antibiotics amoxicillin 500 mg tds, flucloxacillin 500 mg qds, metronidazole 500 mg tds and ceftazidime 500 mg daily and underwent angiography. There was severe narrowing of the popliteal artery and tibioperoneal trunk (Figure 4.21a) and diffuse disease of the calf vessels and very poor flow to the foot. The popliteal artery and tibioperoneal trunk were successfully ballooned to 5 mm (Figure 4.21b, c). However, the foot did not improve and he underwent a right first toe amputation and a right popliteal to dorsalis pedis bypass. Four months later he underwent a right popliteal angioplasty, because Duplex had shown a proximal and distal stenosis to the graft.

One month later, he developed a purulent discharge from the nail bed of the left first toe. He had dilation angioplasty of a left distal popliteal stenosis found on angiography. Within the next three months, he had developed rest pain of the left foot and then developed extensive patches of necrosis on the left foot. He then he had a successful left popliteal to dorsalis pedis bypass. Both feet are healed and remain intact. He receives follow-up care from the Diabetic Foot Clinic, with graft surveillance.

Learning points

- This patient in end stage renal failure with multiple comorbidities nonetheless underwent successful bypasses to both legs for distal disease.

- Distal bypasses provided pulsatile blood flow to both feet.

- Regular surveillance of angioplasty sites and bypass grafts is an essential part of follow-up care.

- Multidisciplinary care can successfully bring these patients through distal bypass.

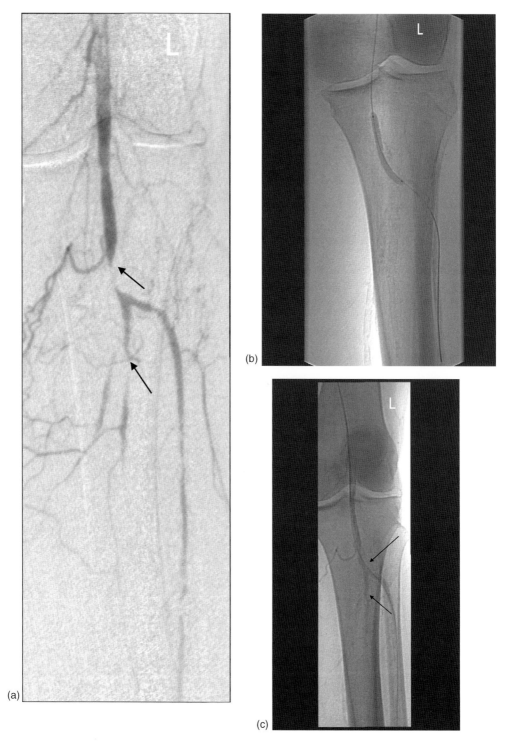

Figure 4.21 (a) Severe narrowing of the popliteal artery and tibioperoneal trunk (arrows). (b) Ballooning of popliteal artery and tibioperoneal trunk. (c) Post angioplasty. Improved flow of popliteal artery and tibioperoneal trunk (arrows).

Case 4.22   Multiple co-morbidities should not preclude bypass

Many grafts need regular "servicing" by the interventional radiologist if they are to maintain good outflow and remain patent long term, and this point is reemphasized in this case.

This man aged 71, with Type 2 diabetes and retinopathy, also had multiple comorbidities, including maculopathy, hypertension, cataracts and ischaemic heart disease. He had a coronary artery bypass graft 3 years previously. When he started haemodialysis, he developed an infection of the left fifth toe and underwent a minor amputation. The amputation site ulcerated, and he then developed further ulceration of the left first toe. Initially, an angiogram was performed, demonstrating occlusion of the anterior tibial and posterior tibial arteries. There was single run-off consisting of the peroneal artery with reconstitution of the plantar arch by a distal posterior tibial artery. He had angioplasty of the peroneal artery but the ulcers did not heal. The patient then underwent a left popliteal to posterior tibial bypass graft. Duplex studies showed the foot being perfused retrogradely by the peroneal artery so he had a jump graft between the posterior tibial and dorsalis pedis one month later. The patient was on haemodialysis throughout.

He then developed problems with the right foot. He had a diseased trifurcation with occlusion of the anterior tibial artery and posterior tibial artery. There was a reconstitution of the dorsalis pedis artery (Figure 4.22a,b). He had an elective popliteal to dorsalis pedis artery graft for ulceration of the first toe of the right foot.

On follow-up, the left graft showed tight stenosis at the proximal anastomosis of the popliteal distal graft and also narrowing in the superficial femoral artery, and the graft was balloon dilated and the superficial femoral artery was also dilated. He was followed up in the Diabetic Foot Clinic. He continues to attend the Diabetic Foot Clinic and the Renal Clinic, and is seen regularly in the Vascular Laboratory.

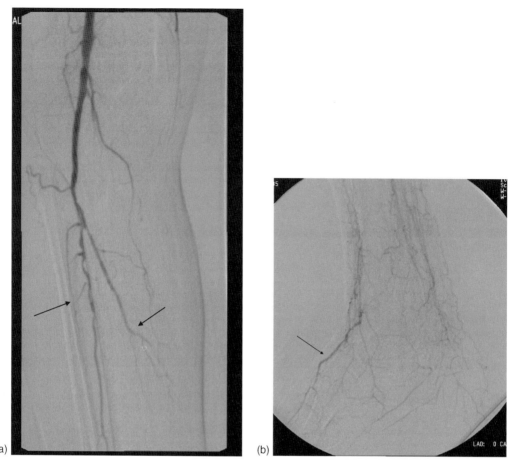

Figure 4.22 (a) Trifurcation, which is diseased with occlusion of the anterior tibial artery and posterior tibial artery (arrows). (b) Reconstitution of the dorsalis pedis artery (arrow) but there is poor opacification of the posterior tibial artery.

Learning points

- A dialysis patient with bilateral bypasses can do well but needed lots of servicing.

- Because of this need for strict surveillance and servicing a multidisciplinary team and access to a vascular laboratory are needed, to ensure close surveillance of wound care, graft function and other health problems.

- During over two decades of managing renal patients with diabetic foot problems we have been aware of their alarming propensity to develop necrosis with great rapidity. We see major pathology in the dialysis patients; however, revascularisation can be performed successfully in these patients. Close liaison between diabetic foot and renal teams is essential.

Index

Diabetic Foot Care: Case Studies in Clinical Management   Alethea Foster and Michael Edmonds
© 2011 John Wiley & Sons, Ltd.